RACING WEIGHT
COOKBOOK

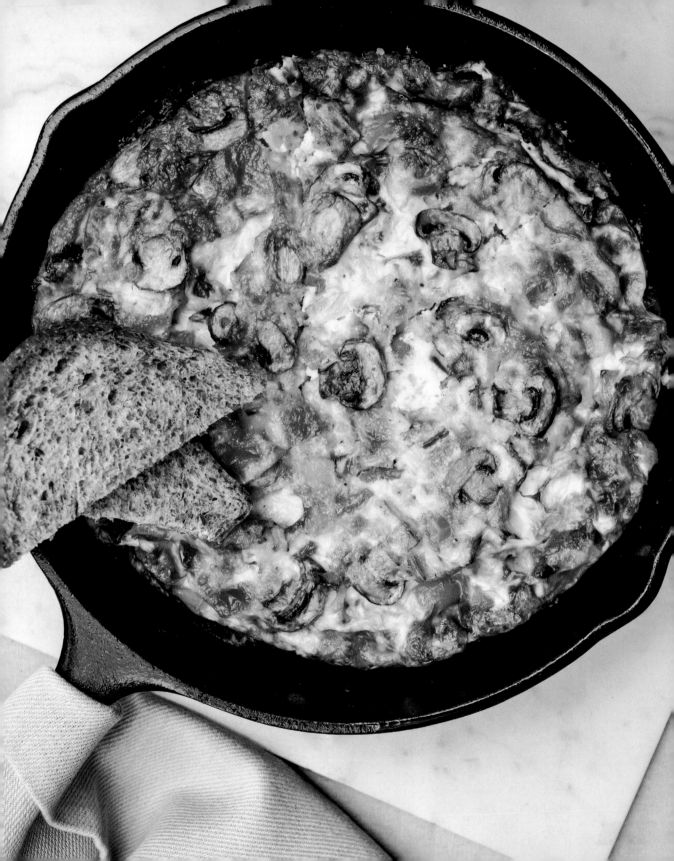

LEAN, LIGHT RECIPES FOR ATHLETES

RACING WEIGHT
COOKBOOK

MATT FITZGERALD
& GEORGIE FEAR

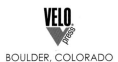

VELO
press

BOULDER, COLORADO

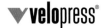

3002 Sterling Circle, Suite 100
Boulder, Colorado 80301-2338 USA
(303) 440-0601 // Fax (303) 444-6788
E-mail velopress@competitorgroup.com

Distributed in the United States and Canada by Ingram Publisher Services

A Cataloging-in-Publication record for this book is available from the Library of Congress.
ISBN 978-1-937715-15-1

For information on purchasing VeloPress books,
please call (800) 811-4210, ext. 2138, or visit www.velopress.com.

This paper meets the requirements of ANSI/NISO Z39.48-1992 (Permanence of Paper).

13 14 15 / 10 9 8 7 6 5 4 3 2 1

CONTENTS

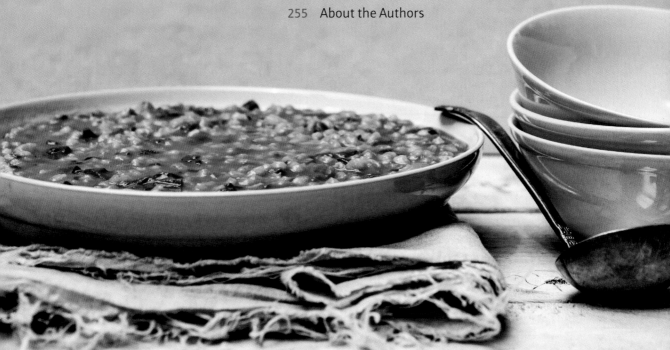

1

THE ATHLETE
WHO DOESN'T COOK

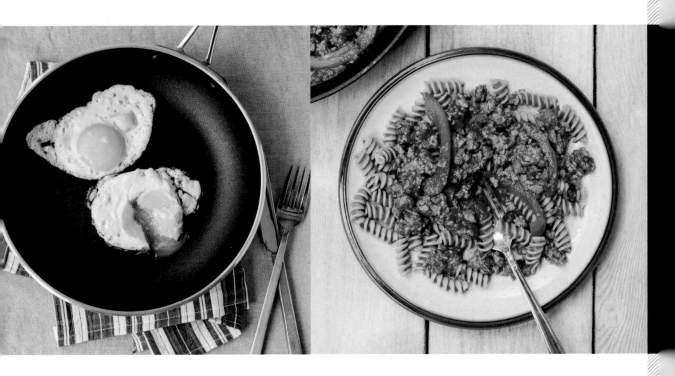

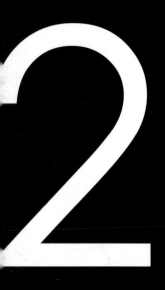

2

RECIPES FOR

THE ATHLETE WITH SOME COOKING EXPERIENCE

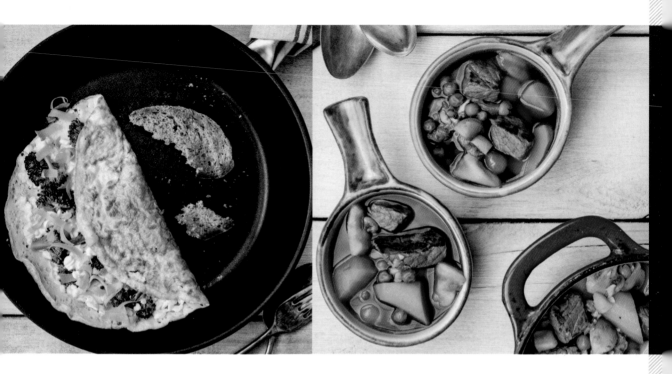

CONCEPTS & TIPS

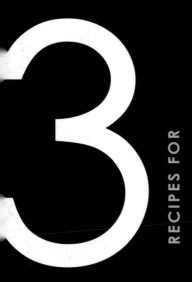

3

RECIPES FOR

THE ATHLETE WHO LOVES TO COOK

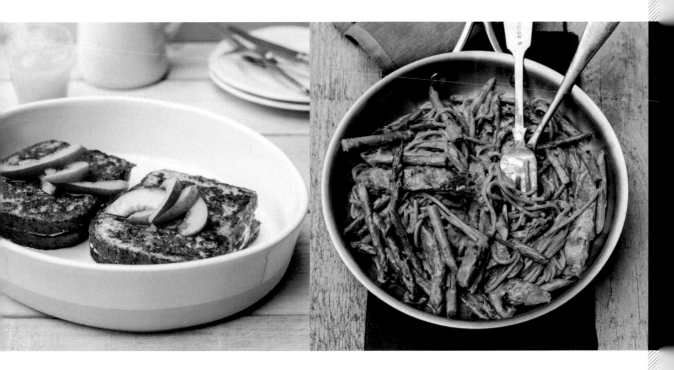

CONCEPTS & TIPS

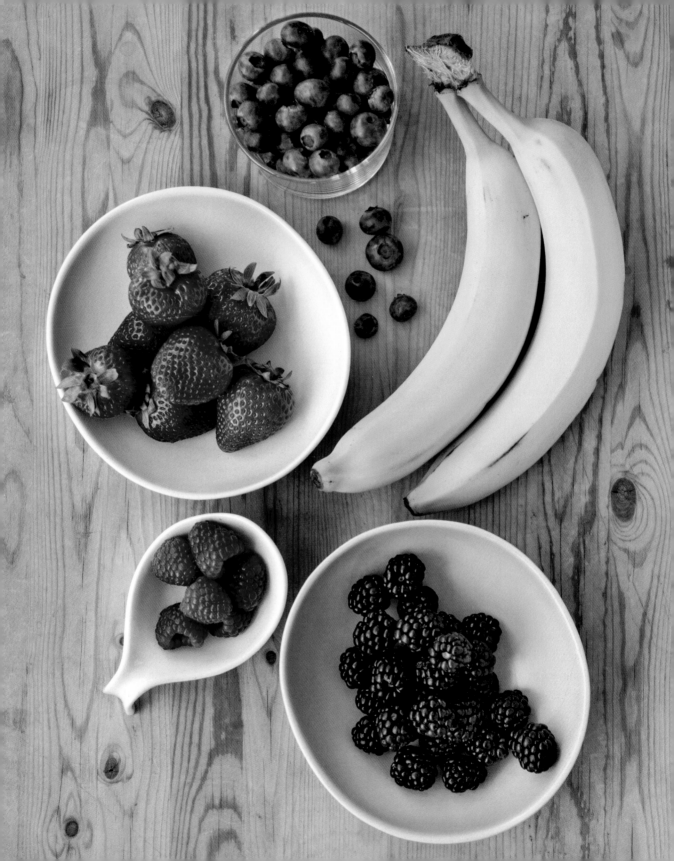

PREFACE

This is not a typical cookbook. It is a cookbook for endurance athletes, who are as different from other categories of eaters as bicycle seats are different from recliners. Cyclists, cross-country skiers, rowers, runners, swimmers, and triathletes have special dietary goals and nutritional needs that are not shared by their nonathlete friends. These unique dietary requirements—especially as they relate to the goal of performance weight management—are thoroughly addressed in my book *Racing Weight: How to Get Lean for Peak Performance.* This cookbook presents original recipes that are consistent with the guidelines offered in that book. Of course, these recipes may also serve as healthy meals for any nonathletes in your household, but they were created especially for athletes like you.

Most cookbooks are written for people who have a preexisting interest in cooking. The *Racing Weight Cookbook* does not presume such an interest because it is intended to enable all endurance athletes, regardless of cooking experience, to feed themselves in a way that conforms to the Racing Weight system. While there are plenty of recipes in the following pages that will appeal to experienced cooks, there are also many that require no special kitchen skills. My highest priority in putting together this book was to ensure that it was useful even to those athletes who generally would rather wash up after dinner than prepare it.

In this regard, my own limited cooking abilities were an advantage. Never drawn to the kitchen, I managed to put off learning how to cook until after I graduated from college. I hadn't been at it very long when I developed persistent stomach pains. Eventually I deduced that the discomfort was caused by pasta sauce. It wasn't that my stomach was especially sensitive to the acids in tomatoes.

The problem, rather, was that I was eating the same meal every single night: spaghetti with ground turkey mixed into Ragú Chunky Gardenstyle Primavera Sauce and a giant stalk of steamed broccoli on the side.

I realized then that in order to be truly healthy, I needed to break out of my comfort zone and learn how to prepare some other kinds of meals. I did not exactly become Wolfgang Puck, but I very slowly added simple meals to my repertoire. I took shortcuts at every opportunity, such as buying canned soups and adding veggies to them instead of making my own soups from scratch. The one thing I refused to do was lower my nutritional standards. Through this combination of laziness and high standards I learned lots of little tricks that enabled me to fuel my body for maximum health and performance without spending more time than I could bear stirring the contents of saucepans. All of the tricks and shortcuts I've picked up over the years are shared in the *Racing Weight Cookbook*. If you can use a can opener, you can use this resource to take control of your diet and reach your optimal racing weight.

Having said this, I hasten to add that cooking is like endurance training (and most other pursuits): The more you put into it, the more you get out of it. Many years ago I had the good fortune to marry a woman whose enthusiasm for cooking has proved infectious. Together we eat a wide variety of enjoyable, healthy meals. This experience has taught me that every endurance athlete should be encouraged to go beyond the basics

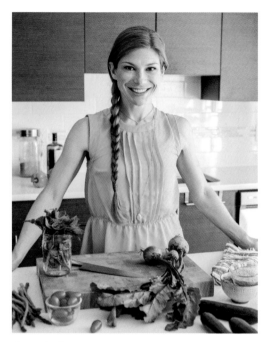

Georgie Fear

and learn how to prepare some meals that offer as much pleasure as they do nutrition.

That's why I did not write this book alone. Georgie Fear is an outstanding cook who creates original meal recipes almost daily for her own enjoyment and to share with the clients she serves as a dietitian and nutrition coach. She is also a fitness fanatic (and a former triathlete and ultrarunner) who understands the special dietary needs of endurance athletes. I've known and admired Georgie for years, and when it came time to choose a collaborator for this book, my list of candidates had only one name on it: hers. All of these recipes were tested and perfected in her kitchen. Thanks to her contributions, the *Racing Weight Cookbook* has as much to offer foodies like her as five-minute cooks like me.

If you're like most people (including most endurance athletes), one of these three phrases accurately describes your relationship with cooking:

1. **I don't cook.**
2. **I have some cooking experience.**
3. **I love to cook!**

The recipes in this book are categorized in three levels that align with these self-descriptions. Level 1 recipes are so simple that even folks who claim they don't cook can put them together without acquiring new skills. Level 2 recipes are a bit more involved but still fall well within the comfort zone of those who have followed basic recipes before. Level 3 recipes are also simple enough to be followed by anyone who can read English but entail a few more steps and some less common ingredients that may be familiar mainly to those who enjoy spending time in the kitchen.

If you haven't cooked before, start with the Level 1 recipes. You can practice the Racing Weight system successfully with these meals alone. Once you've gained a little confidence, you can advance to Level 2 and ultimately to Level 3 recipes. If you're already a little more comfortable in the kitchen, start by drawing from both the Level 1 and Level 2 recipes. You will be ready to advance to Level 3 in no time. And if you're an experienced cook, there are no limitations on which recipes you can use to adhere to the Racing Weight system. Just don't assume that the Level 1 recipes are "too basic" for you. These

meals are no less wholesome than the more sophisticated ones, and even the most avid cook needs a break sometimes.

///

If anyone had told me 20 years ago, when I was fighting stomach pain from eating too much pasta sauce, that one day I would coauthor a cookbook, I would have thought I was hallucinating. Then again, this is not your typical cookbook. It's just the sort of cookbook that I would use (and will use) myself as a runner and triathlete who loves to eat; does not have a lot of time and energy to cook; and is always looking to get leaner, lighter, and faster. I believe that you will discover this to be the perfect cooking resource for you too.

So what are we waiting for? Let's eat!

Matt Fitzgerald

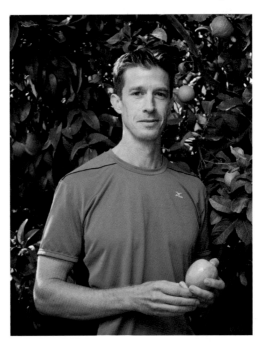

Matt Fitzgerald

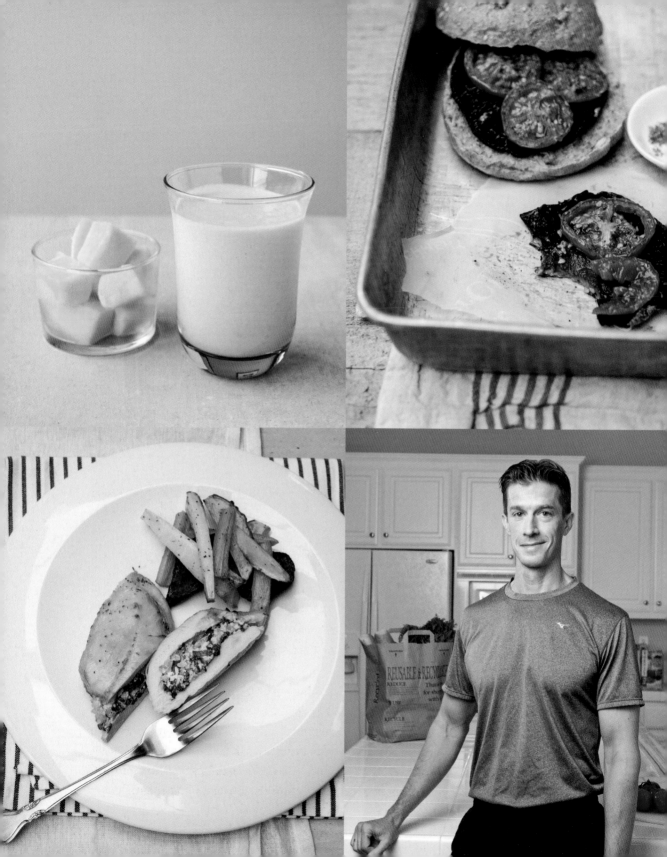

AN INTRODUCTION TO THE RACING WEIGHT PROGRAM

Every endurance athlete has an ideal racing weight. This is defined as the combination of body weight and body fat percentage at which an athlete performs best. Typically athletes perform best when they carry just a little more body fat than the minimum that is required to sustain good health. That's because excess body fat slows athletes down by increasing gravitational resistance, interfering with heat dissipation, and hindering performance in other ways.

Many endurance athletes struggle to reach their racing weight for more or less the same reasons that nonathletes struggle to reach a healthy body weight (for instance, poor food choices and overeating). While the reasons may be the same, the solutions are quite different. Some pursue their racing weight by following popular diets that don't supply enough energy to fuel hard training. I created the Racing Weight program to help athletes reach their racing weight the right way.

The Racing Weight program is a set of six dietary, behavioral, and exercise guidelines designed to help endurance athletes reach their optimal body weight and body composition for racing. All six are widely practiced by the world's most successful endurance athletes and are supported by current science.

1. **Improve your diet quality**
2. **Manage your appetite**
3. **Balance your energy sources**
4. **Monitor yourself**
5. **Time your nutrition**
6. **Train for Racing Weight**

There is nothing radical about the system; it simply works—which means a lot in an environment where all too many athletes are persuaded to try things that don't work. What follows is the essential information you will need to put the program into practice.

1 Improve Your Diet Quality

The single most effective way to get rid of the excess body fat that stands between many endurance athletes and their optimal racing weight is to increase the overall quality of their diet. High-quality foods promote lean body composition and overall good health. Low-quality foods do the opposite. The six categories of high-quality foods are fruits, vegetables (including legumes), whole grains, lean meats and fish, dairy, and nuts and seeds. The four categories of low-quality foods are refined grains, fatty proteins, sweets, and fried foods. Increasing your diet quality is as simple as eating more of the high-quality food types and less of the low-quality food types.

Attaining your optimal racing weight does not require that you eat only high-quality foods and completely avoid low-quality foods. Your diet can be good enough without being perfect. The Diet Quality Score (DQS) is a simple tool that I created to help athletes measure their current diet quality, systematically increase it, and determine when it is indeed good enough.

The DQS is very easy to use. Throughout the course of the day, note each time you eat a food of a given type and look up the DQS value assigned to it in Table 1. (An alternative DQS for vegetarians or vegans is supplied in Table 2.) Note that the points value of a given food type may vary depending on how many times you've already eaten it during the day. This little wrinkle reflects the fact that certain foods aren't as beneficial in large amounts as they are in small amounts. At the end of the day, tally your individual food scores to deter-

TABLE 1 // HOW TO SCORE YOUR DIET QUALITY

| | FOOD TYPE | SERVING NUMBER | | | | | |
		1st	2nd	3rd	4th	5th	6th
HIGH QUALITY	Fruits	2	2	2	1	0	0
	Vegetables	2	2	2	1	0	0
	Whole Grains	2	2	1	0	0	−1
	Lean Meats & Fish*	2	2	1	0	0	−1
	Nuts & Seeds	2	2	1	0	0	−1
	Dairy	1	1	1	0	−1	−2
LOW QUALITY	Refined Grains	−1	−1	−2	−2	−2	−2
	Fatty Proteins	−1	−1	−2	−2	−2	−2
	Sweets	−2	−2	−2	−2	−2	−2
	Fried Foods	−2	−2	−2	−2	−2	−2

* Plant proteins should be scored as vegetables if you are not a vegetarian.

TABLE 2 // HOW TO SCORE VEGETARIAN OR VEGAN DIETS

	FOOD TYPE	SERVING NUMBER					
		1st	2nd	3rd	4th	5th	6th
HIGH QUALITY	Fruits	2	2	2	1	0	0
	Vegetables	2	2	2	1	0	0
	Whole Grains	2	2	1	0	0	−1
	Legumes & Plant Proteins	2	2	1	0	0	−1
	Nuts & Seeds	2	2	1	0	0	−1
	Dairy	1	1	1	0	−1	−2
LOW QUALITY	Refined Grains	−1	−1	−2	−2	−2	−2
	Fatty Proteins	−1	−1	−2	−2	−2	−2
	Sweets	−2	−2	−2	−2	−2	−2
	Fried Foods	−2	−2	−2	−2	−2	−2

mine your overall DQS for the day. If you're not already at your optimal racing weight, find ways to increase your DQS. Keep going until you begin to see the results you seek, and then lock in your DQS at that level, whether it's 16 or 20 or 24 (the maximum DQS is 32). You don't need to hit that mark every day, but you should settle into consistent eating habits that ensure your average DQS equals your target DQS. Be aware that athletes who need to eat more in a day may attain a higher DQS than do those who need to eat less. Don't eat more than you need just to raise your score.

The Diet Quality Score is not a scientific instrument. Use common sense in its application. If you eat half of an apple, count that as half of a fruit serving. If you eat two sandwiches on whole-wheat bread, include two servings of whole grains in your score for that meal. A few slices of pepperoni pizza should

be scored as one serving of refined grains (crust), half a serving of vegetables (tomato sauce), one serving of dairy (cheese), and one serving of fatty meats (pepperoni). Many foods with added sugar should be double-scored. For example, a slice of apple pie should be counted as both a fruit and a sweet.

Although they are high in sugar, honey and maple syrup are not counted as sweets in the Diet Quality Score because they are natural foods like fruits, some of which are also high in sugar. Sugar itself does not necessarily turn a food into a sweet when added to a recipe such as bread, provided the amount of sugar per serving is small. Here's a good rule of thumb to use when scoring baked goods: If it tastes sweet, count it as a sweet (unless it contains honey or maple syrup and no pure sugar). If it doesn't taste sweet, then score it based on the type of flour used.

KEEPING SCORE

There are many small changes you can make every day to take in more nutrients and boost your diet quality. If you use the Diet Quality Score to track what you are eating, you will be able to quickly identify the choices that drag down your score. By finding healthier alternatives to low-quality foods, you can swap a negative score for a neutral or positive score, which makes a surprising difference if you remain consistent. Here are some of our favorite substitutions.

CARBOHYDRATES

+ Carbs are worth counting: too few and your performance will suffer; too many and both performance and weight could be affected. If you've met your carbohydrate needs earlier in the day, choose a lean protein and double up on vegetables for dinner.

PROTEIN

+ Ground turkey or chicken can be a leaner alternative to beef in some recipes.

+ Choose 90 percent lean ground meat instead of more fatty options. When buying solid cuts of beef, look for the words "loin" or "round" on the label to find the leanest cuts. For stew or slow cooker recipes, we like "eye of round," and for grilling "top round" (also called London Broil).

CONDIMENTS

+ Some are better than most. When possible, choose those made with high-quality foods, such as mustard, guacamole, salsa, hummus, and pesto. Try to avoid mayonnaise, ketchup, and barbecue sauce.

+ Choose vinaigrettes rather than creamy dressings for more heart-healthy fats. When you are dining out, ask for salad dressing to be served on the side so you can control the quantity.

DESSERT

+ Try broiled or grilled fruit for dessert. Peaches, plums, and nectarines are especially delicious when grilled or broiled.

+ Instead of eating a pint of frozen yogurt, have a square or two of dark chocolate or a small portion of real ice cream. You'll eat fewer calories, consume less sugar, and may even find that you are more satisfied.

DRINKS

+ Brew homemade iced tea for a good alternative to soda. Bring 4–6 cups water to a boil, turn off the heat, add four teabags, and steep for 10 minutes. Pour into a pitcher and chill. Fruit or mint herbal teas make especially refreshing drinks.

When used sparingly with otherwise high-quality foods, condiments, sauces, and spreads need not be included in a day's DQS. But if you dip your French fries in mayonnaise or smother your pork ribs in barbecue sauce, subtract 1 point from your DQS for the mayo or barbecue sauce in addition to subtracting 2 points for the French fries or ribs.

As for beverages, 100 percent fruit juices may be counted as fruits. Any beverage with added sugar or artificial sweetener is to be classified as a sweet. Don't score your first alcoholic drink of the day if you're female or your first two if you're male, but subtract 2 points from your DQS for any additional drinks. Plain or lightly sweetened coffee or tea has no score. Sports drinks and energy gels also receive no score, provided they are consumed immediately before, during, or after exercise.

Besides prioritizing high-quality foods over low-quality foods in your diet, eating a variety of high-quality food types will boost your DQS and help you reach your racing weight faster. The recipes in this book include a wide variety of high-quality foods and very few low-quality foods. If these meals make up the core of your diet, you will automatically maintain a high DQS. To make things easier, we have included DQS counts for every recipe in the book, but you'll still need to calculate your own score according to what you ate throughout the day using the appropriate table on page 2 or 3.

Remember that there's no "perfect score." If you consistently monitor your weight and performance, your diet will come into focus.

2 Manage Your Appetite

The first thing most of us think of when the topic turns to weight management is overeating and its avoidance. Whether it's high-quality or low-quality, simply eating *too much* food will foil anyone's efforts to lose weight. Because of their high daily energy expenditure, endurance athletes are less likely than are nonathletes to consume more calories than they need. Nonetheless, many athletes eat more than they should because they are subject to the same environmental influences—such as huge portion sizes at restaurants—that induce nonathletes to overeat.

Avoiding overeating does not require that you deny your appetite and go hungry. It merely requires that you *manage* your appetite. Following are eight specific ways to do it.

Learn the difference between belly hunger and head hunger. "Belly hunger" is a set of sensations, including an empty, rumbling stomach and loss of energy, that signals a real, physical need for food. "Head hunger" is a desire to eat for pleasure that occurs in the absence of physical hunger. Attempting to satisfy head hunger is a major cause of overeating. Whenever you experience a desire to eat outside your normal routine, ask yourself whether you are experiencing belly hunger or head hunger. If it's just head hunger, don't eat.

Clean out your kitchen. People are lazy. We are much less likely to eat more than we should or to eat the wrong things when doing so is a hassle. Clearing your refrigerator,

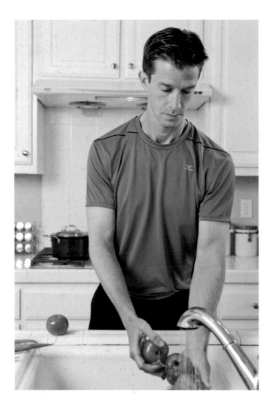

based soups or salads are good appetite spoilers. If you eat a full bowl of soup or an entire salad before you move on to your main dish, you will fill up before you've eaten as much of the main dish as you normally would, and your overall calorie intake will therefore be lower. Several of Georgie's recipes, such as Cauliflower, White Bean & Cheddar Soup (p. 68) or Asparagus & Blue Cheese Soup (p. 143), are well suited to being used this way. Simply adjust the portions to smaller servings if you plan to have soups and salads as appetizers.

Keep healthy foods handy. Remember, people are lazy. Not only are we less likely to eat low-quality foods when they are not convenient, but we are also more likely to eat high-quality foods when they are convenient. Try to keep wholesome snacks close at hand wherever you are. Stash fresh or dried fruit, nuts, or jerky in your desk at the office. Keep a few real-food snack bars such as Georgie's Lemon-Poppy Protein Bars (p. 95; my favorite) in your car and your airplane carry-on bag. If healthy snacks are always within reach, you will use them to manage your appetite instead of going for the usual conveniences of vending machines and fast-food drive-through windows.

At home, where your healthy foods are always in reach, try to also keep them within sight as much as possible. Store refrigerated veggies close to eye level, and keep an attractive bowl stocked with fresh fruit on the kitchen table.

freezer, and pantry of all foods that encourage you to overeat will reduce the number of unnecessary calories you take in.

Use smaller dishes. Research has shown that people tend to eat less without feeling less satisfied when they eat from smaller plates and bowls (such as those featured in many of the photographs in this book). So when you're ready to upgrade your china, be sure to downsize it as well. You'll eat perhaps 10 percent less food in each meal, and you won't miss it.

Spoil your appetite. You may find it easier to avoid overeating if you start each meal by filling some space in your stomach with a food or liquid that has low calorie density. Broth-

EATING JUST ENOUGH

Research suggests that at about age 4, most of us lose touch with the internal signals that, when heeded, reliably govern the amount of food we consume. Instead we allow environmental factors to determine how much we eat, and the result is that we eat too much. Getting back in touch with your body's hunger and satiety signals will help you avoid overeating and reach your optimal racing weight.

To start this process, pay attention to the sensations in your stomach each time you eat. Notice how emptiness gradually transitions into fullness. Through this exercise you will discover that there are many degrees of fullness, ranging from a sort of neutral feeling, where the prior emptiness seems barely covered up, to a feeling of being uncomfortably stuffed. Most of us habitually eat until we are too close to that stuffed feeling.

Experiment with laying down the fork a little earlier each time you eat. If you get really hungry before the next mealtime or if your workouts suffer, you probably cut back too much. Keep eating mindfully and adjusting your quitting point until you discover the degree of fullness that reliably indicates that you've eaten "just enough"—enough to stave off hunger until the next mealtime and to fuel strong workouts but no more.

Once you've locked in this sensation, use it as a guideline going forward. It's a very simple tool, but research has shown that people can lose weight when they make this one change, even if their food choices and activity levels stay the same.

After you've gotten comfortable eating just enough by feel, you can adjust your portion sizes so that you're less likely to have to leave food on the plate. The most challenging part of using this tool is learning to ignore environmental signals to eat more, such as serving sizes in packaged and prepared foods. This includes the serving sizes associated with Georgie's recipes in this book, which you should use only to monitor your nutrient intake and not to govern your food intake. Once you learn how to listen to your body again, you have the perfect tool to help you adapt your portions to meet the changing demands of your training.

Plan for temptation. People are at the greatest risk of overeating when unplanned opportunities to eat tempting low-quality foods catch them by surprise. It's not possible to completely avoid such situations, but you will find it easier to resist temptations if you have a plan for dealing with them before they arise. For example, you might have a standing plan to politely request "just a taste" of any treat that is presented to you by a coworker, friend, or neighbor instead of taking a whole portion of the offered food.

Avoid distracted eating. Much of the over-eating we do takes place in front of television and computer screens and behind wheels. The more you are able to focus on your food while you eat, the less you'll overeat. Even one simple rule, such as not allowing yourself to watch television while eating, could make a difference.

Limit variety. There are two kinds of dietary variety. Good variety is mixing up the foods you eat from day to day to maintain balanced nutrition and keep your diet interesting. Bad variety is including large numbers of differ-ent food items in a single meal. Research has shown that the more food items are included in a meal, the more a person eats. That's why you probably more at buffet-style restaurants than you do elsewhere (and why it's best not to frequent them). So think about ways you can simplify your meals while also remaining focused on incorporating a greater number of high-quality foods in your overall diet.

3 Balance Your Energy Sources

There are three major sources of energy in the diet: carbohydrate, fat, and protein. Endur-ance training increases the body's needs for each of these macronutrients. Research sug-gests that endurance athletes should aim to consume at least 1.2 grams of protein per kilogram of body weight daily (0.55 g/lb.). According to the American College of Sports Medicine, fats should account for at least 20 percent and no more than 35 percent of the calories in an endurance athlete's diet. Carbohydrate needs are more variable and depend on training volume. Table 3 presents recommended carbohydrate intake levels for endurance athletes based on how much train-ing they do.

These carbohydrate recommendations may seem rather high. You can be confident that they are not too high, however. A large body of scientific research has demonstrated that performance in high-volume endurance training programs is compromised when carbohydrate intake is low. In the real world, most elite endurance athletes maintain high-carb diets. The typical elite Ethiopian runner, for example, consumes 10 grams of carbo-hydrate per kilogram of body weight daily (4.5 g/lb.). For a 55-kg (121-lb.) runner, that equates to 550 grams of carbohydrate a day—the amount of carbs in 10 cups of brown rice or 12 cups of whole-wheat pasta. If your cur-rent carbohydrate intake is below the recom-mended level, try increasing it and see if your training doesn't get a boost.

TABLE 3 // HOW MANY CARBS SHOULD ATHLETES EAT?

WEEKLY TRAINING VOLUME	DAILY CARB INTAKE
< 4 hours	2–2.75 g/lb.
5–6 hours	2.75–3.25 g/lb.
7–10 hours	3.25–3.75 g/lb.
11–14 hours	3.75–4 g/lb.
15–19 hours	4–4.5 g/lb.
20–24 hours	4.5–5 g/lb.
> 25 hours	5–5.5 g/lb.

Note: Training intensity affects carbohydrate intake but not nearly to the degree that training volume does, especially for endurance athletes. The recommendations above assume a typical training intensity distribution. Few athletes train at intensities that are so far above or below the average as to render these guidelines inappropriate.

Because carbohydrate needs are so variable, many of Georgie's recipes include options to increase their carbohydrate content. If you train relatively lightly and your carb needs are lower, choose the lower-carb versions of these recipes. If you're in heavy training and your carb needs are higher, choose the higher-carb versions. See additional tips in Meeting Your Carbohydrate Needs (page 14).

4 Monitor Yourself

Successful weight management isn't all about diet. Certain behaviors that have nothing to do with eating can make a difference as well. Research has shown that men and women who have lost weight are less likely to regain it if they weigh themselves frequently. Such self-monitoring techniques enable dieters to catch upticks in their weight in time to prevent them from becoming upward trends.

I recommend that endurance athletes weigh themselves at least once a week and as often as daily. Since optimal racing weight is determined largely by body-fat percentage, I suggest that endurance athletes also measure their body composition (for example, on a home scale with bioelectrical impedance technology) at least once every four weeks. Since the purpose of losing body fat is improved performance, the Racing Weight system also incorporates performance monitoring. Once every four weeks or so (preferably on the days that you measure your body composition), complete some type of standard performance assessment workout. For example, if you're a runner, do a 10K time trial at 90 percent effort. If your performance in these tests gets better, then any associated changes in your weight and body-fat percentage are good.

5 Time Your Nutrition

In the effort to reach your racing weight, it is important that you pay attention not only to what you eat but also to when you eat. Whatever you eat, your body will shed excess fat faster if you take in a majority of your day's calories when your immediate energy needs are greatest and eat little or nothing when those needs are low. The nutrient timing element of the Racing Weight program encompasses seven guidelines for nutrient timing.

Eat early. Your body's energy needs are never greater than when you wake up in the morning. Satisfy those needs by eating some form of breakfast within an hour of leaving bed.

Eat carbs early and protein late. Your breakfast should contain plenty of carbohydrate because your body needs carbs in the morning to replenish liver glycogen stores that have been depleted during the night and to meet the energy demands of the most active part of the day. Your dinner should contain a little less carbohydrate and more protein because at the end of the day the body switches into a biochemical rebuild-and-repair mode, and protein is needed for these processes.

Most of our breakfast recipes are either high in carbohydrate or may be modified to supply an abundance of carbs. The dinner recipes typically contain more protein than the breakfasts do. The 🔴 and 🔵 icons (for high-carb and high-protein) that accompany each recipe will help you select the right ones.

Eat on a consistent schedule. People who eat on a consistent schedule from day to day accumulate less body fat than do people who eat on an erratic schedule, even if their average daily calorie intake is the same. No single eating schedule is right for every athlete, however. Once you find the eating schedule that works best for you, stick to it as consistently as possible.

Eat before exercise. The body's energy needs are greatly elevated during exercise. Therefore, you should start most of your workouts in a well-fueled state. This means you should eat a full meal containing plenty of carbohydrate between four and two hours before your workouts. This is not possible if you train first thing in the morning; in that case, consume a small, carb-rich snack such as a banana before you head out the door.

Eat during exercise. In workouts that are long enough or intense enough to leave you more than moderately fatigued, you will perform better if you take in carbohydrate through a sports drink or energy gels. By performing better in such workouts, you will get extra benefit from them. But you should not take in carbs during all workouts that are long or intense enough to leave you more than moderately fatigued. That's because muscle glycogen depletion stimulates certain physiological adaptations that increase aerobic capacity, and consuming carbs during exercise attenuates glycogen depletion. So you'll want to withhold carbs during roughly half of your workouts that last between one and two hours. Doing this will make those workouts harder, but it will also make you fitter than you would be if you used sports drinks or energy gels as a crutch in all such workouts.

Eat after exercise. After workouts, your body needs carbohydrate to replenish muscle and liver glycogen stores, protein to rebuild damaged muscle tissue, and fluid to rehydrate. The sooner you take in these nutrients after exercise, the more effectively your body will be able to use them. Research has shown that athletes perform better in their next workout when they consume appropriate recovery nutrition within an hour after an initial training session. What's more, athletes who do this habitually actually gain fitness faster because there is a lot of overlap between recovery processes and fitness-building physiological adaptations.

The recipes in this book that work especially well postworkout are identified by a red icon **R** (for recovery).

Minimize eating after dark. During the waking hours, the body's energy needs are lowest between dinnertime and bedtime. People tend to be less active in the evening, and circadian rhythms reduce the functioning of many vital organs at this time. So try to avoid eating again after dinner. It's okay to exempt yourself from this rule if you train heavily and you just can't make it from dinnertime to bedtime without experiencing belly hunger.

///

For more on optimizing your eating schedule and specific guidelines for nutrition before and after workouts, see Healthy Eating for Endurance Athletes (page 16).

6 Train for Racing Weight

Nonathletes often take up exercise for the sole purpose of losing weight. Endurance athletes, by contrast, train for maximum performance in competition. But it happens that the most effective way to train for maximum performance is also the most effective way to train for fat loss. The leanest and most successful endurance athletes follow a high-volume training program in which roughly 80 percent of total training time is spent at lower intensities, 10 percent at moderately high intensity, and 10 percent at high intensity—and so should you.

While the body burns calories faster at higher exercise intensities, you can continue for much longer at lower intensities. Therefore, you'll burn many more total calories without overtaxing your body if you keep your training volume high and the intensity of your workouts fairly low most of the time. Whereas most elite endurance athletes follow the 80/10/10 rule described above, the typical age grouper spends too much time training at a moderate to moderately high intensity. If you are like most age groupers, you need to slightly decrease the intensity of your designated easy workouts in order to free up energy to train more.

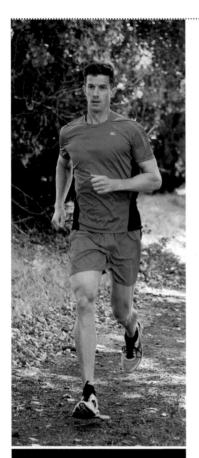

QUICK STARTS

The six-point Racing Weight system is intended to be used when you are actively pursuing peak fitness and your optimal racing weight. It's okay to stray from one or more of the system's guidelines for a few weeks in the off-season. The one time you should not follow the Racing Weight system is when weight loss, rather than peak fitness, is your top priority.

The Racing Weight system is not designed to maximize the rate of fat loss. Rather, it is designed to facilitate slow, steady progress toward optimal racing weight in athletes who are pursuing maximum race fitness. It's not possible to maximize fat loss and fitness gains simultaneously. When fat loss is your top priority, you need to eat and train in ways that do not support the pursuit of peak endurance performance. The most sensible time to make fat loss your top priority is within a four- to eight-week period that immediately precedes the start of focused training for a race or series of races. I refer to such periods as "quick starts" because their purpose is to give athletes a quick start toward their racing weight after an off-season break in which they may have gained a few pounds.

There are three key elements of a properly executed quick start: a moderate daily energy deficit of 300 to 500 calories; increased protein intake (up to 30 percent of total calories); and a training approach that emphasizes weight lifting, fat-burning workouts, and sprint intervals. The high-protein recipes that are most compatible with quick-start dietary guidelines are identified as such with the colored HP icon. Check out my book *Racing Weight Quick Start Guide* for complete guidelines on executing a quick start, including additional high-protein recipes and meal plans.

Quality, Quantity, and Carbohydrate

The Racing Weight program requires that you aim for three basic targets in your daily eating:

+ A Diet Quality Score that's high enough to help you get leaner
+ A total food intake that is determined by a properly managed appetite
+ Adequate carbohydrate to optimally fuel your training, given your racing weight and training volume.

Although these targets are distinct, you will pursue them through the same meals and snacks, so you need to consider all three together when planning your day's eating. Most athletes find that negotiating this balance becomes easier with experience as they settle into dietary habits that hit every target.

When you start the Racing Weight program, focus first on increasing your diet quality. Improving diet quality will help you control your total food intake and will get you close (if not all the way) to your daily carbohydrate intake target. High-quality foods are more satiating than low-quality foods. Thus, as you improve your diet quality your appetite will be satisfied with less food. Many high-quality foods—especially whole grains, fruit, and dairy—are also high in carbohydrate. For this reason, a high-quality diet is likely to provide most if not all of the carbohydrate you need even if you don't actively count carbs. While carbohydrate

needs increase with training volume, so does appetite—so your carb intake will self-adjust as your training increases, and along with it your appetite and your consumption of high-quality foods.

Maintaining high diet quality and eating enough to satisfy your appetite do not guarantee that you will hit your carb intake target, however. I recommend that you count carbs periodically to make sure you're hitting your target. If, after increasing your diet quality, you discover that you're falling short of meeting your daily carb needs, you can easily make up the balance with one or more simple adjustments. For example, you might replace a serving of nuts and seeds with a serving of fruit.

Although not common, there are scenarios in which two of the three basic Racing Weight diet targets come into conflict and you'll need to compromise. As a general rule, when you cannot hit your carbohydrate or DQS target without eating more than your appetite requires, obey your appetite. When you cannot hit your carb intake target without sacrificing DQS points, prioritize your carb intake target. I'll give you a couple of examples.

Suppose you've just eaten dinner on a given day, and you decide to tally up your DQS. When you do, you discover that you're two points shy of your target, so you consider eating a piece of fruit to make up the difference. In this scenario, unless you become hungry before you go to bed, you should not eat the fruit (or anything else). Avoiding over-

MEETING YOUR CARBOHYDRATE NEEDS

Once you figure out just how many grams of carbohydrate you need to take in each day (see Table 3, page 9), you can use Nutrition Facts labels provided on food packages as well as the recipes in this book to see if you are getting enough carbs in your diet. Simply look for "total carbohydrate," taking into account your serving size. *Racing Weight Cookbook* offers you three simple ways to adjust the carb content of your diet:

1 Select recipes that are specifically high-carb or high-protein—use the colored **HC** or **HP** icons for reference.

2 Adjust portion sizes— if you need more carbs, it's likely that you also require more total calories.

3 Supplement recipes with the carb-up options shown in Table 4.

TABLE 4 // EVERYDAY CARB-UP OPTIONS

+ CARBS 15 g	4 oz. fruit juice (100%) 1 cup berries ½ medium baked potato or sweet potato 1 slice whole-grain bread
+ CARBS 30 g	8 oz. fruit juice (100%) 1 large apple or banana 1 medium baked potato or sweet potato 1 whole-grain pita 1 whole-wheat English muffin
+ CARBS 45 g	1 large baked potato or sweet potato 1 cup cooked whole-wheat pasta 1 whole-grain bagel 1 cup cooked brown rice, quinoa, barley, or other whole grain

Because your training volume may vary throughout the year or you may decide to use the Quick Start method prior to a new season of training (see page 12), the recipes in this book can be easily adapted to meet different carbohydrate demands. Some recipes feature specific carb-up tips. For example, you might add brown rice to soup to boost the carbohydrate content. If the lower-carb option better fits your goals, leave out the brown rice.

eating is more important than attaining the highest possible DQS. Smaller athletes and those with lower training loads don't need to eat as much as larger and harder-training athletes. Furthermore, smaller athletes may not have as high a DQS. That doesn't mean their diet is truly of lower quality. As long as you minimize your intake of low-quality foods and eat neither more nor less than enough to satisfy your appetite, your DQS will be what it should be, whatever that number is.

Similarly, if you get to the end of the day and realize you are a few grams shy of your carbohydrate target, again let your appetite rule. Unless you get hungry before bedtime, don't eat any more carbs.

Finally, if there's ever a conflict between your carb target and your DQS, and appetite is not a factor, then give precedence to your carb target. In most cases you should be able to increase your carb intake (if necessary) without lowering your DQS, but there are rare instances in which such a trade-off is almost unavoidable. For example, suppose you are a serious triathlete who maintains a very high training volume and must eat a lot. You're already consuming four servings of fruits and vegetables every day plus three servings each of lean meats and fish, nuts and seeds, whole grains, and dairy. Given this scenario, you may decide to eliminate your third daily serving of lean meats and fish and replace it with a fourth serving of whole grains. This will reduce your DQS

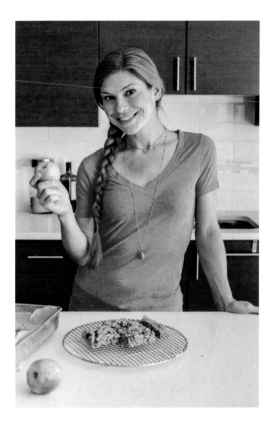

by one point, but you'll probably come out ahead by getting the extra carbs you need to fuel your training.

There is no such thing as a perfect diet. Don't stress yourself out trying to achieve perfection on the Racing Weight program. The goals of maintaining high diet quality, eating the right amount of food, and consuming enough carbs are highly complementary but not absolutely so. You might have to orchestrate a little give-and-take among these goals as you figure out a way to practice the Racing Weight program that works best for you.

HEALTHY EATING FOR ENDURANCE ATHLETES

Everyone eats on some kind of schedule. As an athlete, you need to eat on a schedule that takes into account the timing of your workouts. What follows is information on how to adjust your eating schedule to be more consistent and effective.

◼ Eating Before Exercise

The last meal you eat before a workout must balance two objectives. The primary objective is providing energy for your muscles and nervous system, but in fulfilling this purpose the preworkout meal must also minimize the risk of causing gastrointestinal distress during the workout.

The timing, size, and composition of a preworkout meal influence how well it fulfills its dual purpose. A meal containing plenty of carbohydrate will do the best job of ensuring an adequate supply of energy for the workout. The smaller your meal is and the more time you allow between it and the workout, the less likely it will be to cause uncomfortable stomach sloshing, bloating, or other symptoms during the workout. But if the meal is too small or eaten too long before the workout, its carbohydrate content may be largely used up by the time you start the workout.

TABLE 5 // GUIDELINES FOR PREWORKOUT MEALS

EARLY MORNING	Small, easily digested, high-carb snack such as a banana eaten immediately after waking	+ Banana + Energy gel + Low-fat fruit yogurt
MIDMORNING	Full breakfast with plenty of carbs eaten 3–4 hours before exercise	+ Blueberry-Walnut Pancakes (p. 101) + Pumpkin Oatmeal (p. 102) + Stuffed French Toast (p. 189)
NOON	Small to moderate-sized high-carb snack eaten 2 hours before exercise	+ Energy bar + Tropical Mango Smoothie (p. 44) + Whole-Wheat Fig Bar (p. 181)
LATE AFTERNOON	Full lunch with plenty of carbs eaten 3–4 hours before exercise	+ Garden Minestrone (p. 75) + Roasted Red Pepper & Red Lentil Soup (p. 124) + Quinoa Fried Rice & Wasabi Meatballs (p. 223)
EVENING	Small to moderate-sized dinner eaten 2 hours before exercise	+ Chipotle Chicken Avocado Wrap (p. 64) + Tomato-Basil Soup (p. 153) + Autumn Stuffed Acorn Squash (p. 214)

TABLE 6 // OPTIONS FOR NONSOLID RECOVERY NUTRITION

	SERVING SIZE	CARBO-HYDRATE	PROTEIN
Amy's Organic Lentil Soup	14 oz.	50 g	16 g
Endurox R⁴ All Natural Muscle Recovery Drink	12 oz.	52 g	13 g
Naked Protein Juice Smoothie (no sugar added)	8 oz.	34 g	16 g
Organic Valley Chocolate Reduced Fat Milk	8 oz.	24 g	8 g
Stonyfield Farm Organic Fruit on the Bottom Yogurt	6 oz.	22 g	6 g

The optimal timing, size, and composition of your preworkout meals will depend on when you normally fit your workouts into the day and on how your body responds to different pre-exercise eating patterns, something only experience can teach. Pay attention to how you perform and to how your GI system feels in workouts following meals of different sizes, compositions, and degrees of temporal separation from your workouts. Identify the patterns that work best and then make them habitual.

Table 5 shows some general guidelines for meal patterns that typically work best for workouts performed at different times of the day.

Eating After Exercise

How often do you feel really hungry during a workout? If you're like most athletes, not very often, because exercise suppresses appetite. This effect typically lasts well beyond the workout itself, with hunger returning an hour or more afterward. The more intense the workout is, the longer it is likely to take to feel ready to eat.

The appetite-suppressing effect of exercise tends to thwart athletes' efforts to accelerate recovery through the use of immediate postworkout nutrition. Fortunately, research has shown that semisolids and liquids that are much easier to consume after hard workouts support recovery just as well as solid foods. Remember, the most important nutrients for recovery are carbohydrate for muscle refueling and protein for muscle repair. So if you choose to drink or slurp your postworkout nutrition, be sure to select sources that contain both of these vital nutrients.

In addition to not being hungry, athletes often lack the energy to prepare a meal or are away from home and thus unable to fix food after training. Nonsolid sources of recovery nutrition are sometimes preferable in these circumstances as well. Table 6 shows five convenient options for nonsolid recovery nutrition. Or, with a little preparation, you could enjoy smoothies or bars from this cookbook after your workout.

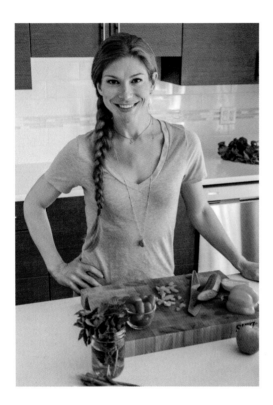

Everyday Eating Habits

As we mentioned earlier, people who eat on a consistent schedule from day to day tend to be leaner than those whose eating schedule is erratic. For this reason you should make a conscious effort to eat your meals and snacks at roughly the same times seven days a week. But this doesn't mean that the same eating schedule is best for everyone. Here are some factors to consider when figuring out your personal eating schedule.

Which comes first: breakfast or exercise? Everyone should eat breakfast. But when you eat breakfast will necessarily depend on whether or not you work out early in the morn-

ing. If you do, eat a light, carb-rich snack after waking and then eat a full breakfast within an hour after completing your workout. If you don't train until later, eat a full breakfast within an hour after getting out of bed.

Try to do the same thing every day—or at least every weekday. Suppose you are a triathlete who wakes up early for masters swim classes on Monday, Wednesday, and Friday mornings. In this case, you might want to wake up early on Tuesday and Thursday to run or ride—even though you don't have to—for the sake of maintaining a consistent eating schedule.

Locking in lunch. Lunch has a way of floating for office workers. On slower days you may be able to duck out for soup and a salad at 11:45. On meeting-packed days it might be 2:00 before you have a chance to eat. Such inconsistency will tend to slow your metabolism and promote fat storage. So do whatever it takes to lock your lunch into the same time every day. Schedule meetings around your lunch hour, pack lunches that you can eat at your desk when necessary, and so forth.

To snack or not to snack. Some endurance athletes need snacks; others don't. If you are smaller and/or train relatively lightly, it is likely that you will get all the energy you need from breakfast, lunch, and dinner. If you are larger and/or train heavily, you may need as many as three snacks each day in addition to three square meals. Once you've determined how many snacks you need daily, plug them into your routine.

Eating on Weekends

It is difficult if not impossible for some endurance athletes to eat on the same schedule on weekends as they do during the week. You may catch up on sleep Saturday and Sunday mornings, making a later breakfast necessary. Or perhaps you do a multihour group bike ride on Saturday morning, making a later lunch necessary that day.

Many people who follow specific dietary rules during the week relax those rules on the weekend. According to research, they pay a price for it. Dieters who succeed in losing weight during the week tend to stop losing weight on Saturday and Sunday, while those who hold steady during the week tend to gain weight on the weekend. It's okay if your weekend eating schedule is a little different from your weekday routine. But at least be sure to maintain your normal diet quality standards on weekends.

In contrast, men and women who maintain the same dietary habits on weekends and weekdays tend to be leaner than average. One simple way to increase your dietary consistency throughout the week is to use the recipes in this book for most of your meals seven days a week. Following are some other tips.

Spread out the drinks. Alcohol tends to promote leanness when consumed in small amounts daily and to do the opposite when consumed in occasional larger doses. So you're better off having a glass of wine every day with dinner than you are teetotaling through the work week and then tying one on Friday night. Sure, there may be fewer total calories in those Friday-night cocktails than there are in seven glasses of wine, but it's not all about math. The benefits of consistency extend beyond the numbers.

Forget about "cheat" meals. Many of us like to reward ourselves for a week of hard work by eating low-quality foods on the weekend. There's nothing wrong with eating a few pieces of fried chicken every now and then, but your food treats should not become a weekend routine. As with alcohol, you're better off allowing yourself to enjoy small amounts of your favorite low-quality foods daily than you are saving them up for the weekend and then going nuts.

Beware the restaurant trap. People are more likely to eat out on weekends, and when people eat out they are more likely to eat low-quality foods (and consume more than one alcoholic drink). The solution to this problem is not necessarily eating out less. Instead, choose restaurants where you know you can get high-quality foods you enjoy—and when you get there, order them. With a little discretion, it's entirely possible to hit the same Diet Quality Score target on days that include a restaurant meal that you aim for on other days.

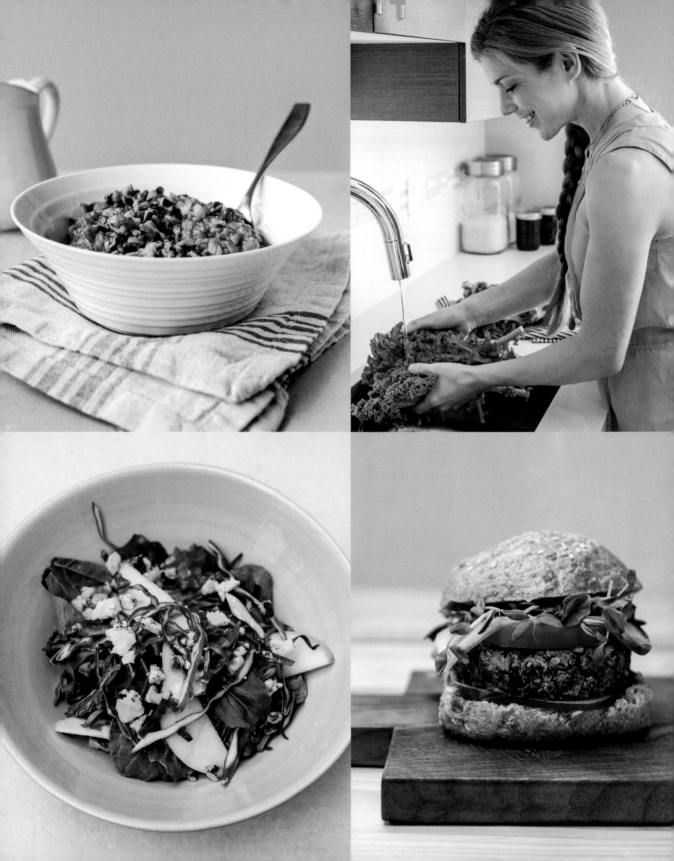

PRACTICAL TIPS
TO GET YOU STARTED

This cookbook was created specifically to help endurance athletes like you put my Racing Weight system into practice. It is intended, therefore, to be used systematically. Of course, you may use it like a regular cookbook if you wish, picking it up once or twice a week when you're in the mood to try something new. But you'll get the most out of it if you base your diet on the recipes and guidelines it contains.

Your first step is to use the Racing Weight system to establish consistent patterns for your diet. Step two is to select meals from this book that enable you to re-create those patterns day by day. Optimal execution of the Racing Weight system does not require that you limit your diet exclusively to these recipes, but the results you seek will come most easily if these meals form the core of what you eat. In order to give you a little extra flexibility, we have included tips for food shopping, eating out, and other practical matters. These tips appear in this section and throughout the book.

The colored icons that accompany each recipe will help you quickly identify the recipes that best match up with your training schedule and individual preferences.

HC HIGH-CARBOHYDRATE
These recipes are especially suitable for athletes with higher carbohydrate needs.

HP HIGH-PROTEIN
These recipes are ideal for quick starts, when you're aiming to get about 30 percent of your daily calories from protein.

R RECOVERY
Have these recipes on hand for postworkout meals and snacks.

V VEGETARIAN
These recipes contain no meat or fish. Note that some but not all vegetarian recipes are vegan (no eggs, dairy, honey, etc.).

FOOD SHOPPING MADE SIMPLE

It goes without saying that in order to prepare all of the great recipes in this book, you must have the necessary ingredients in your kitchen. You won't get very far with the Salmon Cakes with green onion, ginger, and garlic, for example, if you don't have salmon or ginger. The main options for purchasing the stuff you need to make this meal, or any other, are supermarkets (such as Safeway), "big-box" wholesalers (such as Costco or Sam's Club), natural-foods grocers (such as Whole Foods Market), and farmers markets. Weigh the advantages and disadvantages of each venue against your personal needs and priorities to determine the best way to go about stocking your kitchen.

SUPERMARKET

Pros. The big plus of supermarkets is convenience. Chances are there's at least one major supermarket located close to your home. These stores offer the biggest selection and variety of name brands as well as store-brand products, so if you are particular about the brands you buy, the supermarket will be your primary food-shopping venue. Prepackaged or convenience products such as shredded and precut vegetables, already-cooked rotisserie chickens, and salad or olive bars can save you even more time. You can also rely on supermarkets for year-round availability of almost all types of produce.

Cons. Supermarkets provide limited information about the origins of foods other than produce and seafood. For meats and dairy products, you will likely find little information about where and how the animals were raised. Also, supermarkets are filled with tempting processed items (many of them disguised as "health" foods).

TIP *Check the supermarket circular to find out what's on sale. When brand-name foods are marked down, they are sometimes even cheaper than the store brand.*

FARMERS MARKET

Pros. Farmers markets offer the freshest produce, which is often organic and/or sourced from local farmers. If you enjoy knowing the story behind your food, there's nothing better than a farmers market, where you may meet the people who produced the food on display. It's a fun way to shop if you have a little extra time and a great opportunity for kids to learn about and appreciate their food.

Cons. The prices can range from inexpensive to exorbitant, depending on the market, season, and products. Expect limited selection at certain times of the year, and keep in mind that no matter how much you rely on farmers markets to stock your refrigerator, you will find yourself making other trips to pick up items on your list that the market does not have (canned beans or baking powder, for example). Generally, there are no convenience options such as frozen vegetables at these venues.

TIP *Find out what's in season. Don't expect to find lots of flavorful tomatoes during a February trip to the farmers market. Plan your menu accordingly.*

WHOLESALER

Pros. Grocery wholesalers always compete on price. Use them to save money on nonperishable foods that you use frequently. While these stores aren't known for health food, they do offer some high-quality foods in convenient forms and at lower prices than you can find elsewhere. For example, they often have single-serving packages of nuts (since vending-machine suppliers use these stores), which are not available in supermarkets. I like to hit my local big-box store once in a while to stock up on single-serving bags of pistachios and almonds.

Cons. Oh, those tempting samples! (Steer clear; they are usually processed items that aren't healthy for you.) Having bigger boxes and bags of food at home leads us to eat more, so you're fighting an uphill battle when you have a 10-pound jug of cashews. Try to avoid buying larger amounts of perishable items (vegetables, fruit, cheese) than you'll use before they expire. Finally, wholesale stores

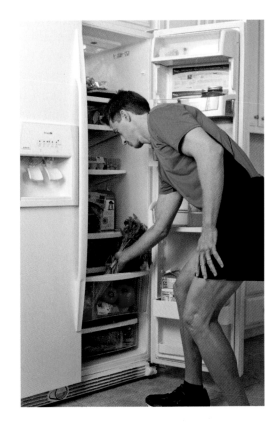

have limited variety of brands, flavors, and high-quality foods.

TIP *Determine how much storage space you have and what you need. Draw up a list before you leave home and stick to it.*

NATURAL-FOODS GROCER

Pros. Natural-foods grocery stores tend to be the best places to shop for an abundance of high-quality foods. Their fresh produce is often organic and local. Many specialty items are available for those on restricted diets due to gluten intolerance, allergies, or other special needs. You are also likely to find a wide selection of healthy premade foods that can be used to replace a meal out if you need to eat and are short on time (or patience). Many natural-foods grocers apply ethical standards to the sourcing of their seafood and meat—for example, Whole Foods Market sells only seafood that meets specific standards for sustainability.

Cons. Expect to pay a lot more money for an equivalent amount of food at a natural-foods grocer than you do almost anywhere else. Beware the "health halo"—organic cookies are still cookies, loaded with sugar and not the most healthful choice. Just because a food is organic, free-range, low-fat, low-carb, or gluten-free doesn't mean it is healthy.

TIP *Get a clear sense of your personal dietary priorities so you don't get seduced by marketing hype or think that you must buy gluten-free pasta because you happen to see gluten-free pasta. It's also helpful to know what kinds of organic produce are most worth spending a little extra money for. We recommend that you arm yourself with the Environmental Working Group's lists of the Dirty Dozen and Clean Fifteen, which are updated every year.*

ONLINE INGREDIENT SOURCES

Depending on where you live, some ingredients may not be available at your local store. Here are some of our favorite food sites for the ingredients you will need to make Georgie's recipes.

Natural Foods, Whole Grains, and Legumes

+ Bob's Red Mill
www.bobsredmill.com
Barley, beans, chickpea flour, lentils, rolled oats, millet, oat bran, pearl barley, quinoa, wheat berries, wheat bran, whole-grain spelt flour

+ Hodgson Mill
www.hodgsonmill.com
Whole-wheat couscous, whole-wheat pasta

Dried Fruit, Nuts, and Seeds

+ Nuts.com
Almonds, apricots, chia seeds, figs, ground flaxseed, nut butter, pecans, pistachios, raisins, walnuts

Gluten-Free and Allergen-Free Baking Mixes

+ Authentic Foods
www.glutenfree-supermarket.com

+ The Gluten-Free Mall
www.celiac.com/glutenfreemall/

Spices, Herbs, Extracts, and Salts

+ Savory Spice Shop
www.savoryspiceshop.com
Cardamom, coconut extract, lemon extract, macadamia-nut oil, onion flakes

COOKING MADE SIMPLE

Training for endurance sports is time consuming. By precooking proteins and whole grains, you can put together a healthy meal faster. In the recipes, "fast-fix" ingredients are highlighted as _cooked_. Follow the cooking instructions in the chart below and on page 27 so you can take advantage of these fast fixes. Some frozen foods are also highlighted as fast-fix ingredients because they save you prep work.

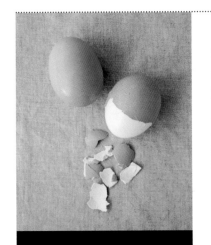

PREPARING PRECOOKED PROTEINS

Cook up a big batch of chicken, beef, or eggs on the weekend in just 15–30 minutes, and enjoy fast-fix meals throughout the week. Lean meats are great additions to pasta sauces, salads, and soups.

CHICKEN BREASTS	Season boneless, skinless chicken breasts with salt and pepper. Bake on a foil-lined sheet for 20 minutes at 400 degrees F. Slice and freeze or refrigerate for up to a week. Bone-in chicken breasts taste great and are cheaper, but you'll need to cook them longer, about 30 minutes. Whenever you cook poultry, it's a good idea to use a thermometer to make sure the center reaches 165 degrees F. Use cooked chicken in Chipotle Chicken Avocado Wrap (p. 64), One-Pot Quinoa, Chicken & Veggies (p. 85), and Curried Chicken Salad with Pistachios (p. 206).
EXTRA-LEAN GROUND BEEF	Brown the meat in a skillet, drain the fat, and refrigerate for up to a week or freeze. Use cooked ground beef in Tomato & Beef Florentine Soup (p. 63), Beefy Stuffed Poblanos (p. 127), and Beef-Vegetable Ragu over Spaghetti Squash (p. 157).
HARD-BOILED EGGS	Place a dozen eggs in a pot with enough cold water to cover by 1–2 inches. Cover and bring to a full rolling boil, then turn off the heat. Let the covered pot sit for 12 minutes, then put the eggs into cold water to stop the cooking. Refrigerate for up to a week. (Note that older eggs are easier to peel than fresh ones.) Use hard-boiled eggs alongside breakfast, as a postworkout snack, or atop salads.

BUYING **READY-TO-EAT PROTEINS**

Ready-to-eat proteins are somewhat more expensive and may contain additives and extra sodium. When you simply don't have the time, here are some tips to help you find high-quality ingredients.

ROTISSERIE CHICKEN

+ It's best to remove the skin to help keep fat grams in check. While dark meat contains slightly more fat than does light meat, it also provides more iron, which is important to athletes. Chop up leftover meat and freeze in 1-cup portions to add to soups, stews, and cooked grains. You can also use rotisserie chicken in our Roasted Chicken and Mushroom Quinoa recipe (pp. 237–238).

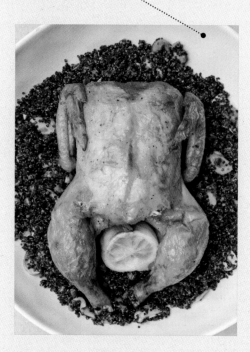

SEAFOOD

+ When buying canned tuna, salmon, and shellfish, choose items canned in water without added oil. Choose chunk-light tuna instead of solid white tuna for less mercury.

+ Look for precooked shrimp in the frozen-foods section. For the shrimp lowest in environmental contaminants, choose shrimp from the United States over varieties sourced from Southeast Asia.

DELI MEATS

+ For filling healthy sandwiches with lean protein, pick up all-natural turkey breast or chicken breast from the deli. If you can view the ingredients, choose deli meats without added nitrates or nitrites.

WHERE ELSE TO LOOK

+ Pick up cottage cheese, Greek yogurt, and cheese in the dairy section. All are excellent sources of protein. You may even find already cooked (and peeled) hard-boiled eggs.

+ Canned beans can also help you meet your protein needs. Simply drain and rinse before adding to soups and salads.

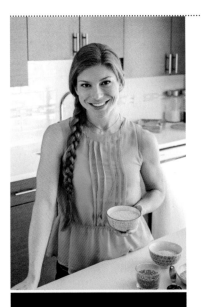

PRECOOKING
WHOLE GRAINS

Adding whole grains to your diet sounds great, but not if it means 45–60 minutes of boiling time before every meal. Cook grains in big batches and refrigerate for up to four days or freeze for long-term storage. Serve as a hot cereal with milk, toss with a green salad, or warm with seasonings for an easy side dish.

Start by rinsing whole grains with cold water. The rest is as easy as boiling water. There are countless varieties, but these are our favorites.

BARLEY	Boil 1 cup barley (or pearl barley) with 3 cups water for 45 minutes. Drain any excess water.	Quick-cooking barley cooks in 10–12 minutes. Follow package directions.
BROWN RICE	Bring 1 cup rice and 2½ cups water or broth to a boil. Turn heat to low and simmer, covered, until tender and most of the liquid has been absorbed, 40–50 minutes. Let stand 5 minutes, then fluff with a fork.	Quick-cooking and instant brown rice cook in 5–15 minutes. Follow package directions.
MILLET	Boil 1 cup millet and 4 cups water for 25–35 minutes.	///
QUINOA	Bring 2 cups water to a boil; add 1 cup quinoa. Turn heat to low and simmer, covered, until the liquid has been absorbed, 15–20 minutes. Fluff with a fork.	Quinoa is a naturally quick-cooking grain.
WHEAT BERRIES	Boil 1 cup wheat berries with 3 cups cold water for 60 minutes. Drain any excess water.	///

THE GIFT OF LEFTOVERS

Cooking just enough to eat one meal at a time works beautifully if you have lots of time on your hands. For 99 percent of us, however, leftovers are a welcome convenience. Most of the recipes in this book make 2–4 servings. You might need two servings just to fuel your training, but there will undoubtedly be times that you have extra food on your hands. Follow these simple guidelines to better enjoy your leftovers.

Planning for leftovers. If you are cooking for two, choose or adapt recipes to serve 4–8. Don't make so many portions of one dish that you have to eat the same thing for a week. Naturally, you'll get sick of it, and some of it will probably spoil.

To double a recipe, double all the ingredients except for the spices, herbs, and salt. With these ingredients, use 1.5 times the original amount. You can always add more seasoning to taste.

Storing and reheating leftovers. Toting home-cooked leftovers to work saves you cash and helps you maintain a high-quality diet. Whenever possible, store your food in glass containers, especially if you intend to reheat it in the same container. Plastic containers that are designated as BPA-free are also fine, but transfer your food to another dish before microwaving. Don't reuse plastic containers such as yogurt or cottage-cheese tubs—the plastic can leach chemicals into your food. Never microwave Styrofoam containers.

To defrost frozen leftovers quickly, use the defrost setting on your microwave and rotate the plate a few times during the process, especially if your microwave doesn't have a turntable. This helps the food thaw out evenly. You can also defrost food for 12–24 hours in the refrigerator. Be sure to put a plate underneath it because there is likely to be some water runoff.

Heat leftovers to an internal temperature of 165 degrees F. A digital food thermometer is a good tool for making sure your leftovers are ready to eat.

///

Be sure to eat your leftovers within three or four days. Most refrigerated foods take longer to spoil, but they lose flavor (and sometimes texture) first. If you want to make big batches of food, refrigerate only what you can eat in two or three days. Freeze the rest for later rediscovery. Soups and stews are great for this. Divide a double batch of chili into thirds and freeze two of them. For more tips, see A Well-Stocked Freezer (page 203).

THE ATHLETE
WHO DOESN'T COOK

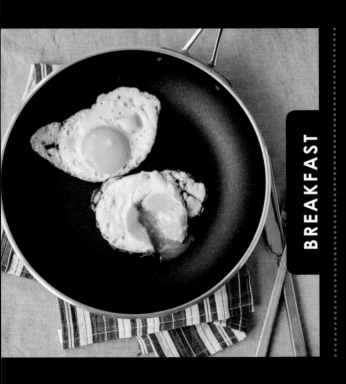

BREAKFAST }

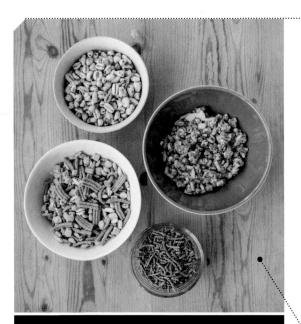

Cold cereal is one of the most popular breakfast foods among endurance athletes. What's not to love? It's ready in an instant, makes no mess, and tastes good. It also can be the foundation of a balanced meal if you select your cereal wisely and add a few choice ingredients to fill in any nutritional gaps.

BREAKFAST CEREAL
DONE RIGHT

PICK A WHOLESOME VARIETY

Select a cereal that lists whole grains as the first ingredient (look for words such as *whole wheat*, *whole oats*, and *whole corn*). Check the Nutrition Facts panel for the amount of sugar per serving, and pick a cereal with less than 8 grams of sugar. If it contains dried fruit, it should ideally be less than 10 grams of sugar per serving. Look for at least 3 grams of fiber.

MIND YOUR SERVING SIZE

Dense breakfast cereals such as granola pack lots of carbs into a small serving volume, often only ¼ or ⅓ cup. Fill your bowl carelessly and you might eat four or more servings, which is likely more calories than you need. To enjoy a bigger serving with fewer calories, fill your bowl with a lower-calorie puffed cereal, flakes, or O's and top it off with granola and muesli.

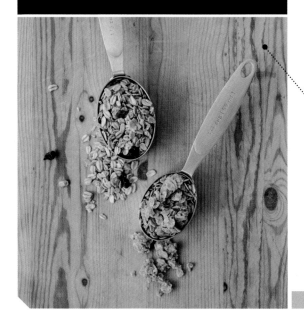

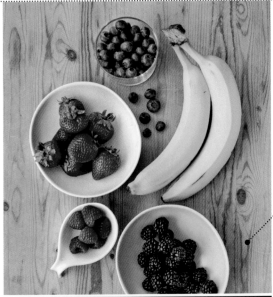

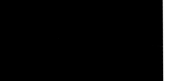

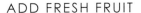

ADD FRESH FRUIT

While cereal is rich in carbohydrates and often fortified with vitamins and minerals, it can't replicate the phytochemicals and health-promoting antioxidants found in fresh produce. Because of its lower caloric density, fruit will help you remain satisfied longer, which in turn will help you in managing your weight. Sliced banana, blueberries, or strawberries add flavor to cereal and improve its Diet Quality Score.

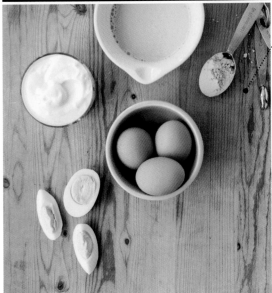

BOOST PROTEIN

Aim for at least 15 grams of total protein in your bowl to curb your appetite. One cup of milk provides 8 grams of protein. Nondairy milks such as almond and soy typically have less protein. A few cereals such as Kashi GOLEAN are fortified with soy protein, but most contain fewer than 5 grams per serving. You can add protein by substituting Greek yogurt for milk (15 g per cup), eating a hard-boiled egg on the side (6 g), or stirring 1–2 tablespoons of vanilla protein powder into milk before pouring it onto your cereal (5–10 g).

WINNER'S CIRCLE YOGURT

No time to cook? That's no excuse for skipping breakfast. A base of plain yogurt provides protein and calcium. Add whole-grain cereal, an important source of complex carbohydrates and fiber. Top it off with fruit for sweetness and flavor and nuts or seeds for minerals, healthy fat, and a good crunch.

PLAIN YOGURT	Try Greek yogurt for higher protein.
WHOLE-GRAIN CEREAL	Original or Multigrain Cheerios, Kashi GOLEAN, Fiber One, Total Whole Grain, or Wheaties
FRUIT	Strawberries, blueberries, raspberries, bananas, or peaches
NUTS	Almonds, walnuts, or pecans
SEEDS	Chia, ground flaxseed, or pumpkin seeds

Start with a bowl of yogurt and add your favorite things for a high-quality breakfast.

If you like to mix it all together but want the cereal to stay crunchy, stir the nuts, seeds, and fruit into your yogurt, then add the cereal on top.

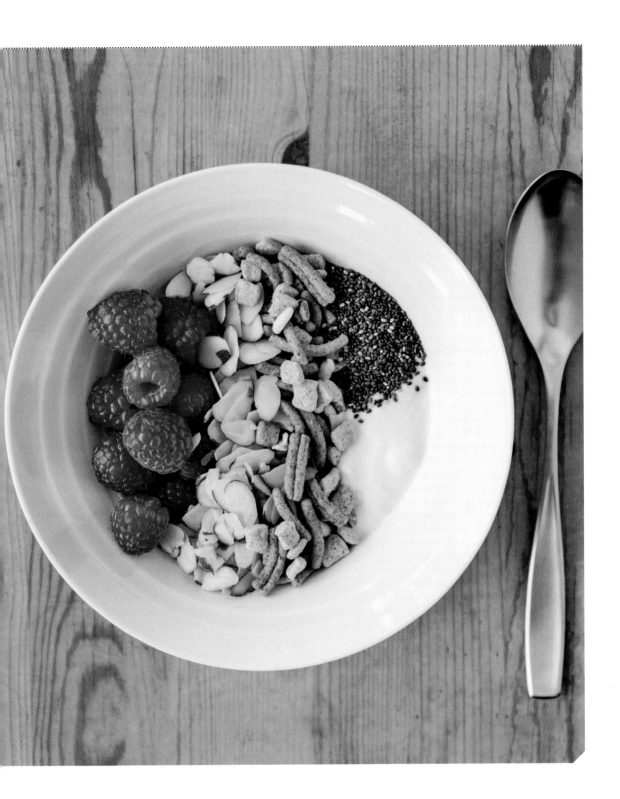

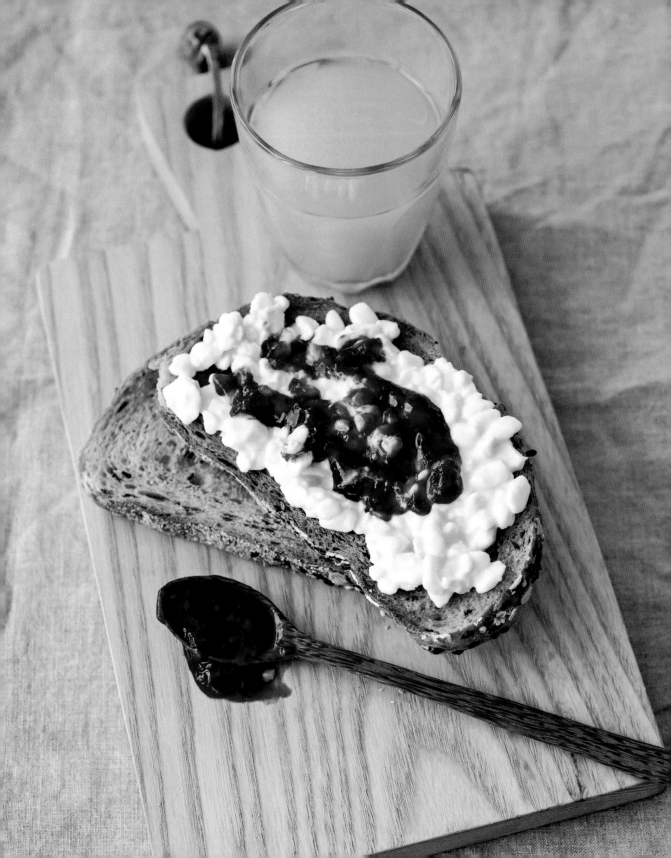

TOAST WITH COTTAGE CHEESE & RASPBERRY PRESERVES

1 SERVING // 5 MINUTES

- 2 slices whole-wheat bread
- ½ cup 2% cottage cheese
- 1 teaspoon all-fruit raspberry preserves

1 Toast bread. Spread each slice with cottage cheese, and top with preserves.

Per serving: 283 calories, 6 g fat, 38 g total carbohydrate, 6 g dietary fiber, 22 g protein

A glass of fresh orange juice will give your DQS a nice boost.

HOW TO KNOW IT'S 100% WHOLE GRAIN

The bread aisle can present a dizzying array of options. Here are four easy steps to picking the right loaf (or buns, bagels, tortillas, etc.):

1. Read the ingredients list. The ingredients are listed by weight, so the first few ingredients are the most important.

2. The first ingredient should be *whole-wheat grain flour* or *whole-wheat flour*. If you see *enriched wheat flour* or simply *wheat flour*, put it back on the shelf. Those are simply other names for white flour.

3. Don't settle for less than 100%. Most bread is made with a mixture of whole-wheat flour and less nutritious white flour. Even if the first ingredient is whole-wheat flour, scan the rest of the ingredients to ensure that white flour doesn't appear later.

4. Once you've got a truly 100% whole-grain loaf, check the Nutrition Facts panel for the amount of sugar—you want no more than 2 grams per slice.

DQS COUNT (per serving)   WHOLE GRAINS 1   DAIRY 1

PEANUT-BUTTER GRANOLA

6 SERVINGS (¼ CUP) // 20 MINUTES

It is surprisingly easy to make granola. This recipe calls for just a few ingredients that you are likely to already have on hand. Sprinkle granola atop Greek yogurt and add your favorite fruit for a no-cook meal that provides healthy fats, whole grains, fiber, and protein.

3 tablespoons smooth natural peanut butter

3 tablespoons honey

¼ teaspoon vanilla extract

¼ teaspoon salt

1 cup rolled oats (also called old-fashioned oats)

1 Preheat oven to 300 degrees F. Line a baking sheet with parchment paper.

2 In a medium bowl, combine peanut butter, honey, vanilla, and salt, and stir to mix. Heat in the microwave for 20 seconds if peanut butter doesn't melt and mix in easily.

3 Add oats to the bowl, and gently fold to stir them in. Scoop mixture onto lined baking sheet and spread out. Small clumps will form.

4 Bake for 10 minutes, then turn off the oven (leaving the baking sheet inside) and allow granola to cool completely with the oven door slightly open. It will get crunchy as it cools.

Makes 1½ cups.

Per serving: 135 calories, 5 g fat, 19 g total carbohydrate, 2 g dietary fiber, 4 g protein

DQS COUNT (per serving)   WHOLE GRAINS   ½

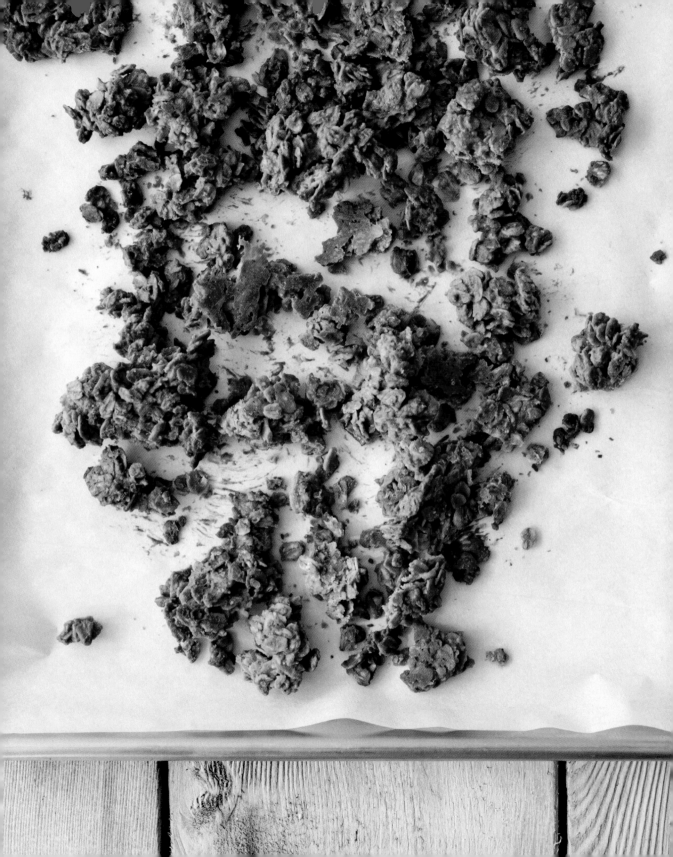

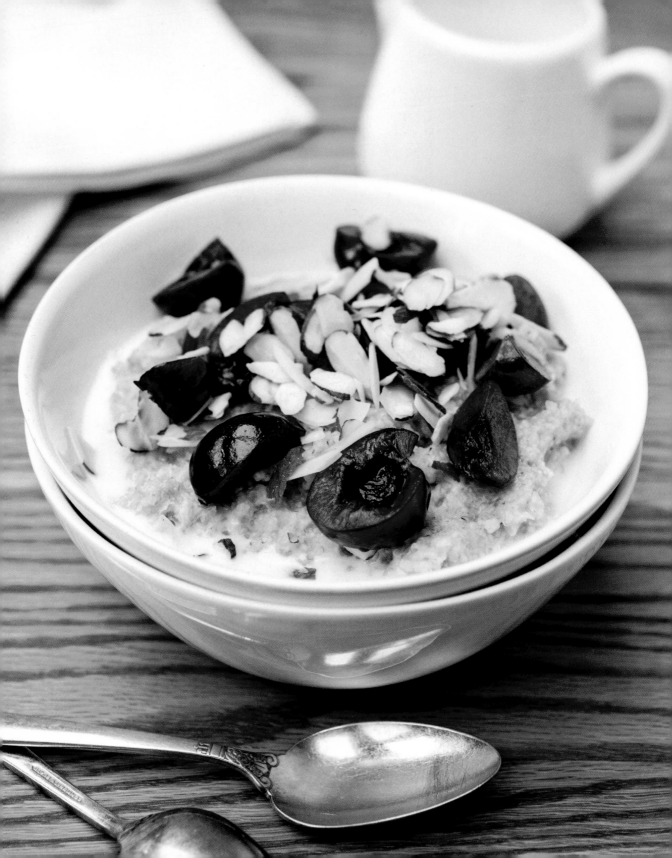

OAT BRAN WITH CHERRIES & ALMONDS

2 SERVINGS // 15 MINUTES

3 cups water

1½ cups oat bran

pinch of salt

2 teaspoons vanilla extract

2 teaspoons sugar

2 cups fresh or frozen cherries

2 tablespoons (½ oz.) almonds, slivered

milk (optional)

1 In a saucepan, bring water to a boil over medium-high heat. Add oat bran and cook uncovered until the mixture begins to thicken, 5–10 minutes. Stir periodically to keep oat bran from sticking to the pan.

2 While oat bran is cooking, cut each cherry in half and remove pit with a paring knife.

3 Season oat bran with salt, vanilla, and sugar and stir to blend. Remove from heat and divide between two bowls. Top with cherries and almonds and a splash of your favorite milk, if desired.

Per serving: 422 calories, 10 g fat, 74 g total carbohydrate, 13 g dietary fiber, 15 g protein

Save time by combining water, oat bran, salt, vanilla, and sugar in a microwave-safe bowl. Microwave for 90 seconds, stir, and microwave for an additional 90 seconds. Let rest a few minutes before topping and serving.

DQS COUNT (per serving)   FRUITS 1   WHOLE GRAINS 1   NUTS & SEEDS 1

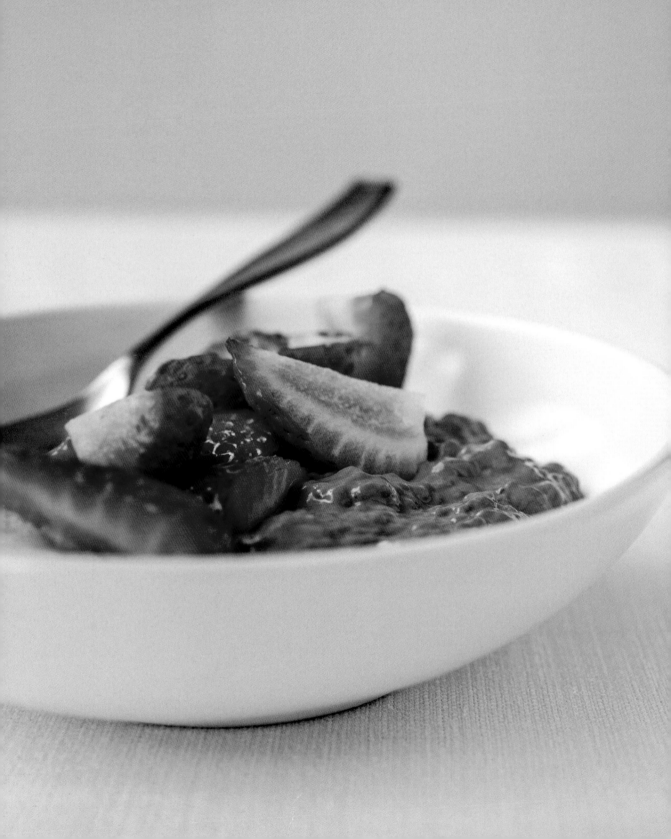

CHOCOLATE CHIA POWER PUDDING

1 SERVING // 5 MINUTES PLUS 20 MINUTES TO CHILL

Chia seeds are a great way to add healthy fats, iron, and fiber to your diet. The seeds absorb liquid and thicken into a delicious pudding. This is a great alternative breakfast if you're tired of cereal but don't want to make anything more elaborate.

1 serving chocolate protein powder

¾ cup unsweetened almond milk, divided

2 tablespoons chia seeds

1 cup strawberries, sliced

1 Combine protein powder with ¼ cup almond milk in a bowl and stir until smooth.

2 Add remaining ½ cup almond milk and chia seeds and stir well.

3 Refrigerate for 20 minutes to let pudding thicken. Top with sliced strawberries.

Per serving: 325 calories, 13 g fat, 33 g total carbohydrate, 17 g dietary fiber, 26 g protein

Leaner Living MRP is our favorite brand of protein powder for taste, smooth mixing, and the highest-quality ingredients.

DQS COUNT (per serving)   FRUITS 1   NUTS & SEEDS 1

TROPICAL MANGO ELECTROLYTE BOOSTER

1 SERVING // 5 MINUTES

This smoothie's refreshing citrus and mango flavors aren't the only perk. It contains valuable electrolytes such as sodium and potassium plus vitamin C, carbohydrate, and protein to help you recover optimally from long, hard training sessions.

1 cup water

1½ cups (5 oz.) _frozen_ mango chunks

2 tablespoons lemon-lime hydration mix

1 serving vanilla protein powder

1 Combine all ingredients in a blender and process until smooth.

Per serving: 358 calories, 4 g fat, 60 g total carbohydrate, 9 g dietary fiber, 21 g protein

DQS COUNT (per serving)   FRUITS 1

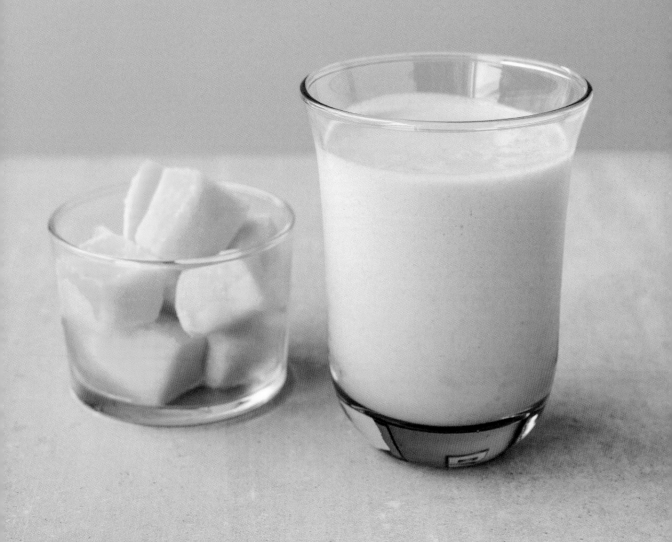

EGGS
3 WAYS

 TIP

Whenever you work with a nonstick pan, as we recommend for all three of these dishes, make sure to use a heat-resistant silicone, plastic, or rubber spatula. Metal utensils can damage the pan's nonstick coating.

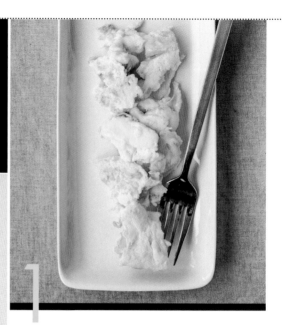

1

SCRAMBLED EGGS
1 SERVING // 5 MINUTES

  2 eggs
  2 tablespoons milk
     pinch of salt
     pinch of pepper
  ½ teaspoon extra-virgin olive oil

Whisk eggs, milk, salt, and pepper in a bowl with a wire whisk or fork.

Place oil in a nonstick skillet over medium heat for 60–90 seconds. A drop of water should sizzle in the pan when hot enough.

Pour in eggs and reduce heat to low. As eggs begin to set, gently move a spatula around the pan to form large, soft curds. Cook until eggs are no longer runny but not dry.

Per serving: 178 calories, 12 g fat, 0 g total carbohydrate, 0 g dietary fiber, 13 g protein

DQS COUNT (per serving)

| LEAN MEATS & FISH | 1 |

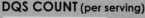

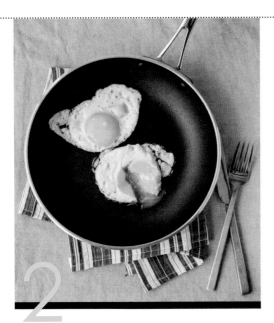

FRIED EGGS

1 SERVING // 5–7 MINUTES

    2 teaspoons extra-virgin olive oil
    2 eggs
       salt and pepper

Place oil in a nonstick skillet over medium heat for 60–90 seconds. A drop of water should sizzle in the pan when hot enough.

Crack one egg into a small bowl, then slide egg into the pan. Repeat with other egg.

Let eggs cook for 3 minutes, then cover for 30 seconds to cook whites. For runny yolks, remove eggs immediately. For set yolks, turn off burner and leave in covered pan for 1–2 minutes more.

Season with salt and pepper to taste.

Per serving: 140 calories, 9 g fat, 0 g total carbohydrate, 0 g dietary fiber, 12 g protein

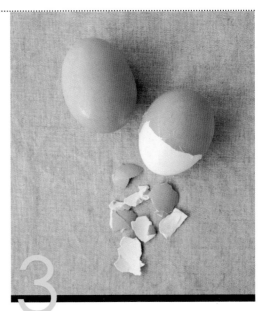

HARD-BOILED EGGS

3 SERVINGS (2 EGGS) // 15 MINUTES

    6 eggs
       water

Place eggs in a pot and add cold water to submerge by 1–2 inches. Cover pot and bring to a rolling boil over high heat. Turn off heat and let the covered pot sit for 12 minutes.

Transfer eggs into cold water to stop the cooking.

Store hard-boiled eggs in the refrigerator for up to 1 week.

Per serving: 220 calories, 18 g fat, 0 g total carbohydrate, 0 g dietary fiber, 12 g protein

 TIP

Hard-boiled eggs are easier to peel after some time in the refrigerator.

NUT BUTTER & BANANA TOAST

1 SERVING // 5 MINUTES HC R V

2 slices whole-wheat bread

1 banana

2 tablespoons natural almond butter or other nut butter

1 Toast bread. Spread each slice with 1 tablespoon nut butter, and top with sliced banana.

Per serving: 455 calories, 18 g fat, 59 g total carbohydrate, 9 g dietary fiber, 15 g protein

PEANUT BUTTER AND OTHER NUT BUTTERS

The most healthful nut butters are made without any added sugar, sweeteners, or hydrogenated oils. Look for natural nut butters made from only nuts or nuts and salt. Don't be fooled into buying reduced-fat peanut butter, as it offers negligible calorie savings thanks to added sugar. Besides, peanut and other nut butters are sources of healthy fats that are good for your heart and cholesterol levels.

If you've never tried a nut butter that isn't peanut butter, you're missing out. Try almond, cashew, or NuttZo multinut butter (made from a blend of seven nuts and seeds). For those with nut allergies, sunflower-seed butter and pumpkin-seed butter are great alternatives to nut butters in recipes.

DQS COUNT (per serving)   FRUITS 1   WHOLE GRAINS 1   NUTS & SEEDS ½

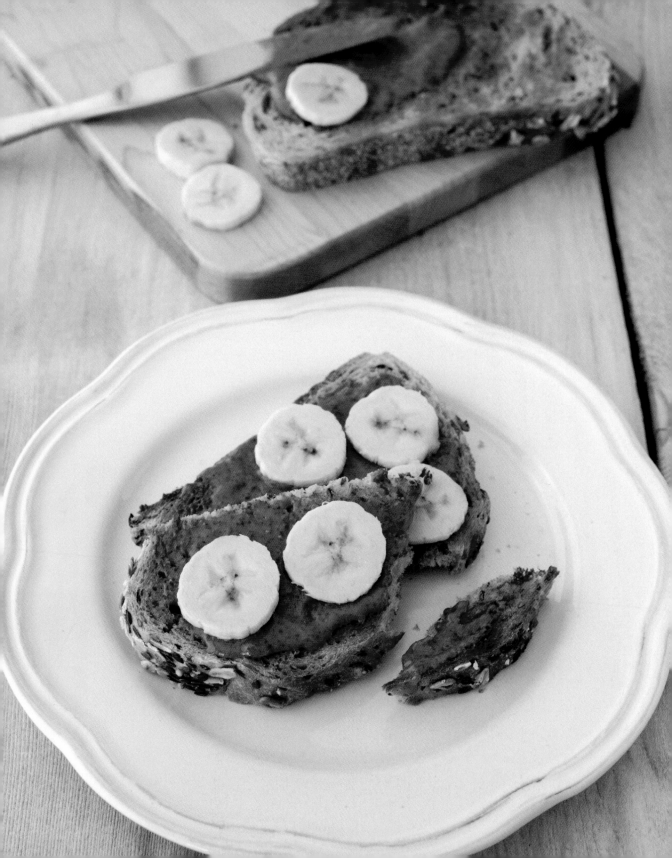

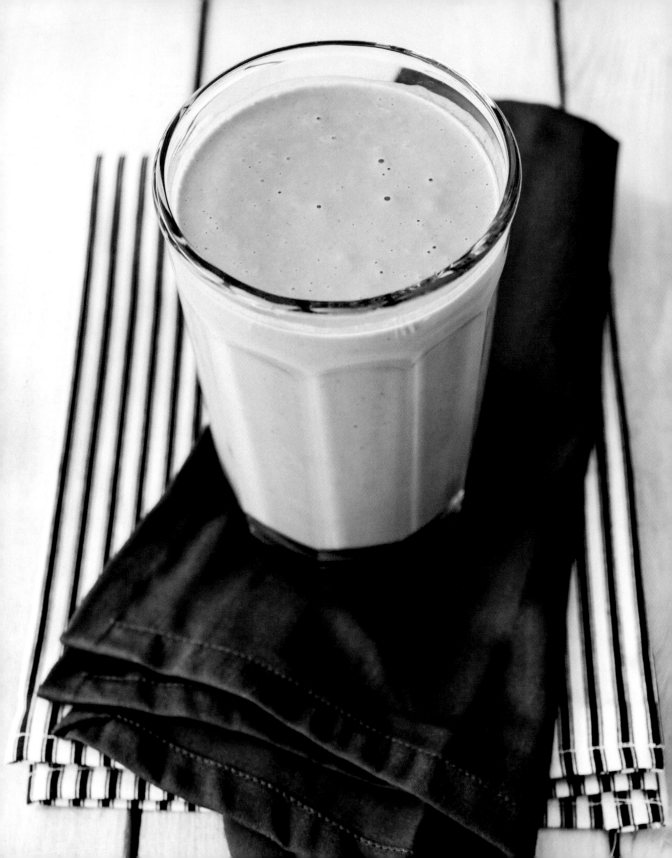

CHOCOLATE PEANUT-BUTTER BANANA SHAKE

1 SERVING // 5 MINUTES (R) (V)

If you have no time to eat a meal following a workout, here's a well-balanced option. Thanks to heart-healthy fats from the nut butter and lots of protein, this shake will keep you satisfied for hours.

1 cup water

1 frozen banana

1 tablespoon smooth natural peanut butter

1 serving chocolate protein powder

1 Combine all ingredients in a blender and process until smooth.

Per serving: 375 calories, 12 g fat, 40 g total carbohydrate, 10 g dietary fiber, 26 g protein

PERFECTLY RIPE BANANAS

Bananas are often a staple for athletes. If you purchase a bunch of six bananas, they will all ripen within a two- to three-day period. Chances are you will not be able to eat all six bananas as soon as they are ripe! To have perfectly ripe bananas any day of the week, pick up singles with varying degrees of ripeness. Buy a couple that are ready to eat in the next day or so, a couple that are slightly green at the ends (which will be ready in three or four days), and a couple that are slightly green throughout (which will be perfect in about a week). In the event that you do end up with overripe bananas, just peel them and freeze them in plastic bags—they will be great for pancakes or smoothies.

DQS COUNT (per serving)   FRUITS 1   NUTS & SEEDS ½

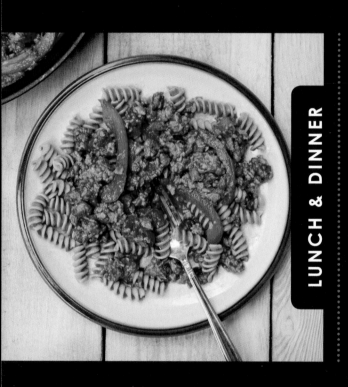

}

1

THE ATHLETE
WHO DOESN'T COOK

5-MINUTE BURRITO

Once you've ventured into the frozen-foods aisle, it's easy to think there's no hope for a nutritious meal. Not so! A good-quality frozen meal or burrito can be made even better with some quick additions. Start with a product containing whole-food ingredients that you can pronounce, and with no trans fats. We recommend brands such as Amy's Kitchen or Kashi, which make great-tasting and healthy all-natural frozen foods. Try to find a product with at least 15 grams of protein.

We made this burrito into a completely nutritious meal in just 5 minutes.

1 Amy's bean and cheese burrito

2 plum tomatoes

½ avocado

2 tablespoons salsa

Remove plastic wrap from burrito. Wrap burrito loosely in paper towel, place in microwave, and heat for 2–2½ minutes or until hot.

While burrito is cooking, quarter tomatoes and cut avocado in half. Scoop avocado flesh out of the skin with a spoon. (Refrigerate leftover avocado in plastic bag.)

When burrito is heated through, transfer it to the plate and add tomatoes, avocado, and salsa.

Per serving: 460 calories, 20 g fat, 60 g total carbohydrate, 13 g dietary fiber, 13 g protein

TIP

If your favorite burrito is short on protein, consider adding a hard-boiled egg, canned tuna, or cottage cheese as a side to bump up the protein.

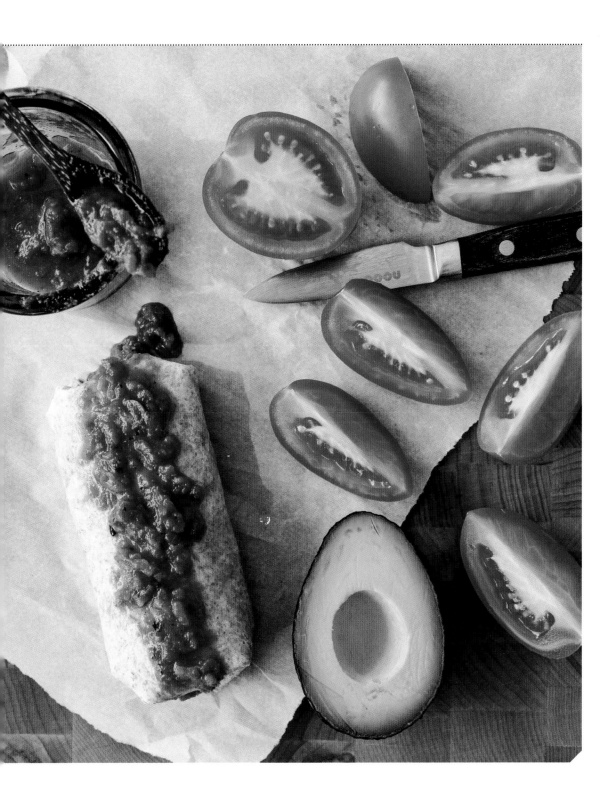

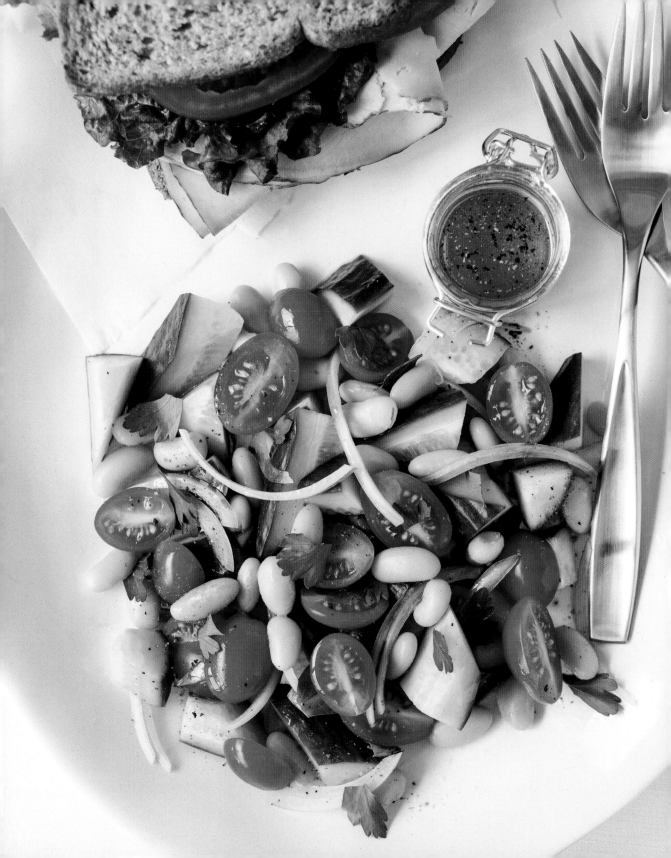

WHITE BEAN, TOMATO & CUCUMBER SALAD

2 SERVINGS // 10 MINUTES PLUS 30 MINUTES TO CHILL

This delicious high-fiber salad can be a delightful change of pace from lettuce-based salads. Allowing it to sit for at least 30 minutes before enjoying helps the flavors meld, and it's even better the second day.

1 15-ounce can white beans (Great Northern or cannellini), rinsed and drained

1 pint cherry or grape tomatoes, quartered

1 large cucumber, chopped (seeded and peeled, if desired)

⅔ cup red onion, chopped

⅔ cup fresh parsley, chopped

¼ cup white or red wine vinegar

2 tablespoons extra-virgin olive oil

¼ teaspoon salt

⅛ teaspoon black pepper

1 Combine all ingredients in a large mixing bowl and stir gently to combine. Refrigerate until ready to serve.

Store leftovers in refrigerator for up to 5 days.

Per serving: 379 calories, 16 g fat, 45 g total carbohydrate, 15 g dietary fiber, 16 g protein

When buying canned tomatoes and beans, look for varieties without added salt.

DQS COUNT (per serving)   VEGETABLES 2 (1 legumes)

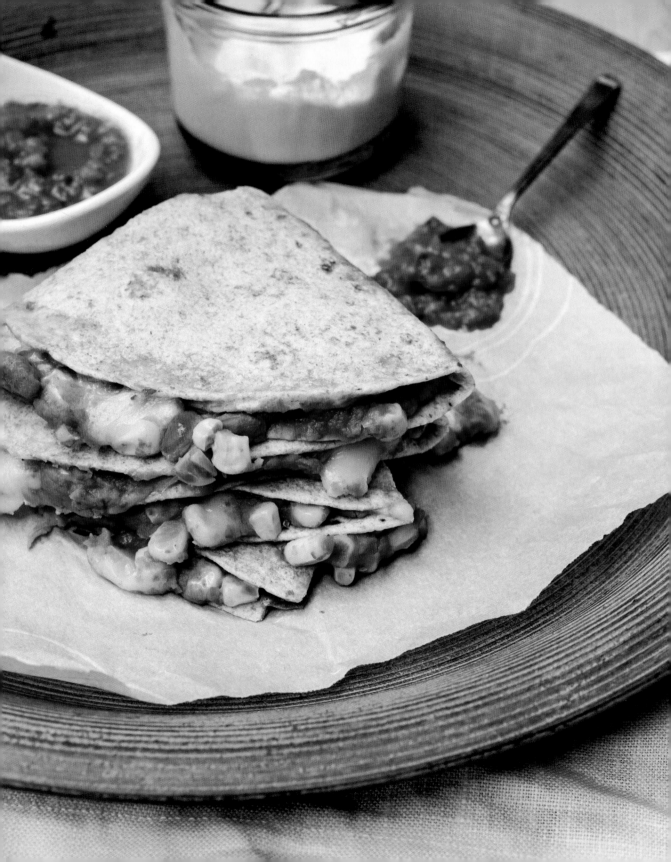

BEAN, CORN & CHEESE QUESADILLA

1 SERVING // 10 MINUTES (HC) (R) (V)

Improve on a classic snack food by incorporating high-fiber whole grains, refried beans with protein-rich cheese, and Greek yogurt instead of sour cream. Use string cheese and frozen corn to save time.

⅓ cup _frozen_ whole-kernel corn

½ cup canned refried beans

1 string cheese, chopped

1 large whole-wheat or sprouted-grain tortilla

¼ cup salsa

¼ cup plain Greek yogurt

1 Thaw corn in a small bowl in the microwave for 30 seconds. Mix in refried beans and cheese.

2 Gently spread the beans, corn, and cheese mixture over half the tortilla, folding the other half over the top.

3 Place tortilla in a large nonstick skillet over medium heat. Cook until the bottom of the tortilla becomes golden brown—use a spatula to lift it and take a peek. Flip over and cook until the other side is also golden brown and contents are heated through.

4 Slide quesadilla onto cutting board and cut into four wedges. Top each wedge with salsa and Greek yogurt.

Per serving: 450 calories, 10 g fat, 61 g total carbohydrate, 11 g dietary fiber, 28 g protein

DQS COUNT (per serving)   VEGETABLES 1½ (½ legumes)   WHOLE GRAINS 1   DAIRY 1

BLACK-BEAN BURGER FAJITA SALAD

1 SERVING // 15 MINUTES Ⓥ

Fajita vegetables, black beans, avocado, and cheese make this salad a Tex-Mex delight without the extra fat that a burrito or fajita entrée typically entails. Frozen black-bean burgers will save you time.

cooking spray

1 *frozen* black-bean burger

¾ cup (3 oz.) bell-pepper strips (frozen or fresh)

¼ cup onion, chopped

¼ cup mushrooms, sliced

½ teaspoon salt

½ teaspoon chipotle powder or chili powder

2 cups fresh baby spinach, loosely packed

¼ avocado, cubed

2 tablespoons (½ oz.) shredded cheddar cheese

1 Coat a large nonstick skillet with cooking spray and bring to medium heat. Place the frozen black-bean burger in the skillet and cook for 3 minutes on each side.

2 At the same time, add peppers, onion, and mushrooms to pan. Season vegetables lightly with salt and chipotle powder. Cook until vegetables are soft, about 5 minutes, and remove from heat.

3 Place spinach on a plate and top with cooked vegetables and cubed avocado. Coarsely chop burger and place on top of salad. Finish with shredded cheese, and serve with whole-wheat tortilla, if desired.

Per serving: 296 calories, 15 g fat, 27 g total carbohydrate, 12 g dietary fiber, 18 g protein

+ CARBS Add a whole-wheat tortilla for 49 g total carbohydrate.

DQS COUNT (per serving) VEGETABLES 2 (1 legumes) DAIRY ½

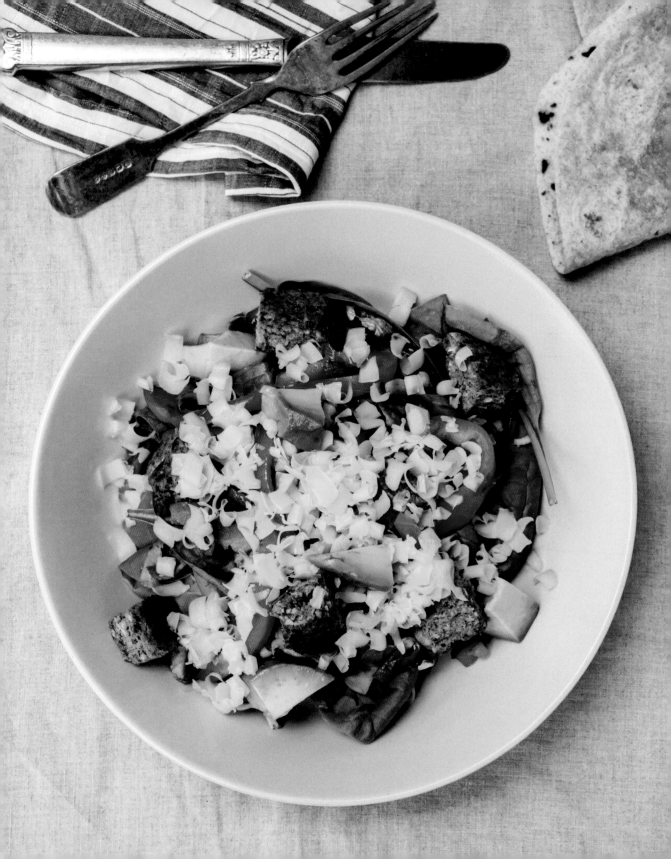

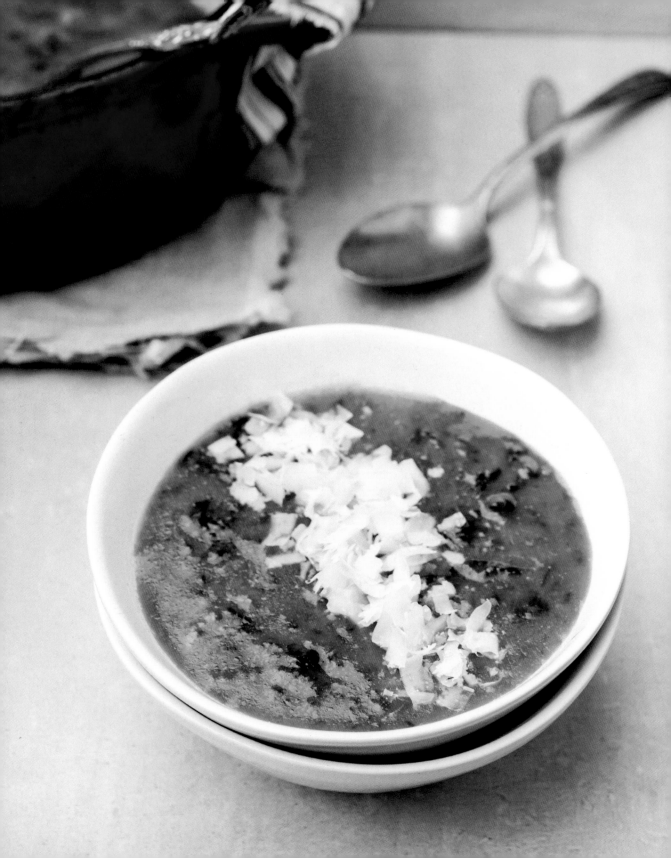

TOMATO & BEEF FLORENTINE SOUP

2 SERVINGS // 15 MINUTES

Jazz up your canned soup with leftover chicken or beef, extra vegetables, and herbs. Keep in mind that canned soups typically have more than enough salt, but you might want to add black pepper, cayenne pepper, or a dash of hot sauce.

- 10 ounces *frozen* cut leaf spinach
- 2 10¾-ounce cans condensed tomato soup
- 2 cans (2½ c.) water
- 1 cup *cooked* extra-lean ground beef
- 1 teaspoon dried basil
  black pepper
- 2 tablespoons Parmesan or feta cheese

1 Place frozen spinach in a bowl and defrost in microwave for 3 minutes or until mostly thawed. Squeeze out excess liquid over the sink.

2 In a saucepan over medium heat, warm tomato soup and water.

3 Stir in cooked beef, spinach, and basil, and cook over medium heat for about 10 minutes or until hot. Season with pepper to taste. Ladle into two large bowls and top with cheese.

Per serving: 510 calories, 10 g fat, 61 g total carbohydrate, 2 g dietary fiber, 32 g protein

DQS COUNT (per serving) VEGETABLES 2 LEAN MEATS & FISH 1 DAIRY ½

CHIPOTLE CHICKEN AVOCADO WRAP

1 SERVING // 20 MINUTES

- 8 ounces boneless, skinless chicken breast or tenders
- ½ teaspoon chipotle powder
- ½ teaspoon salt
- ½ red onion (grill before slicing)
- 2 10-inch whole-grain tortillas
- ½ cup (5½ oz.) roasted red peppers from a jar
- ½ avocado, sliced

1 Preheat indoor or outdoor grill. Season chicken on both sides with chipotle powder and salt.

2 Place chicken and onion on grill and cook for 8–10 minutes or until chicken is fully cooked and onion is soft. Slice grilled onion when it's cool enough to handle.

3 Place a tortilla on each plate and top each with half the roasted red peppers and avocado. Divide cooked chicken and onions evenly and fold or wrap to close.

Per serving: 410 calories, 13 g fat, 43 g total carbohydrate, 5 g dietary fiber, 33 g protein

DQS COUNT (per serving) VEGETABLES 1   WHOLE GRAINS 1   LEAN MEATS & FISH 1

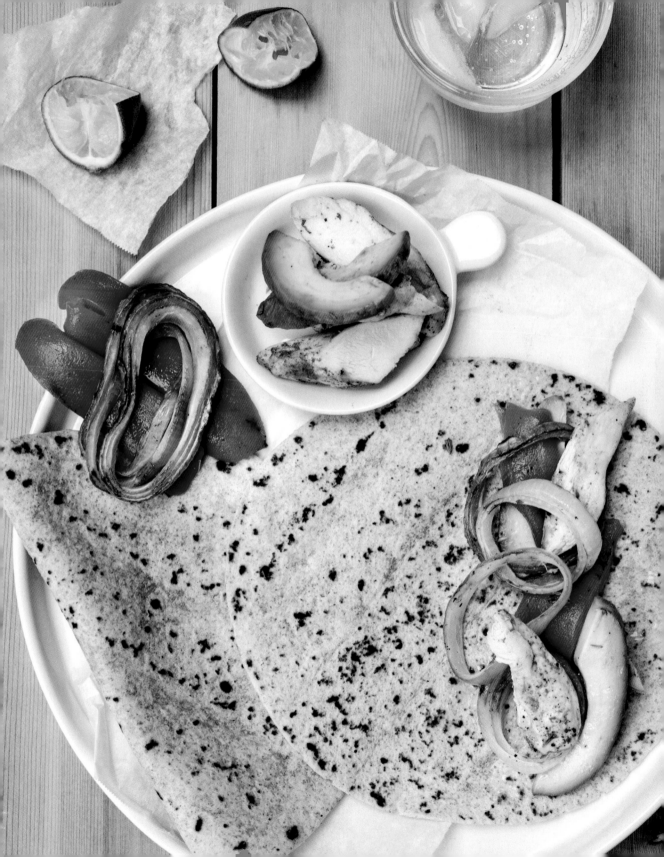

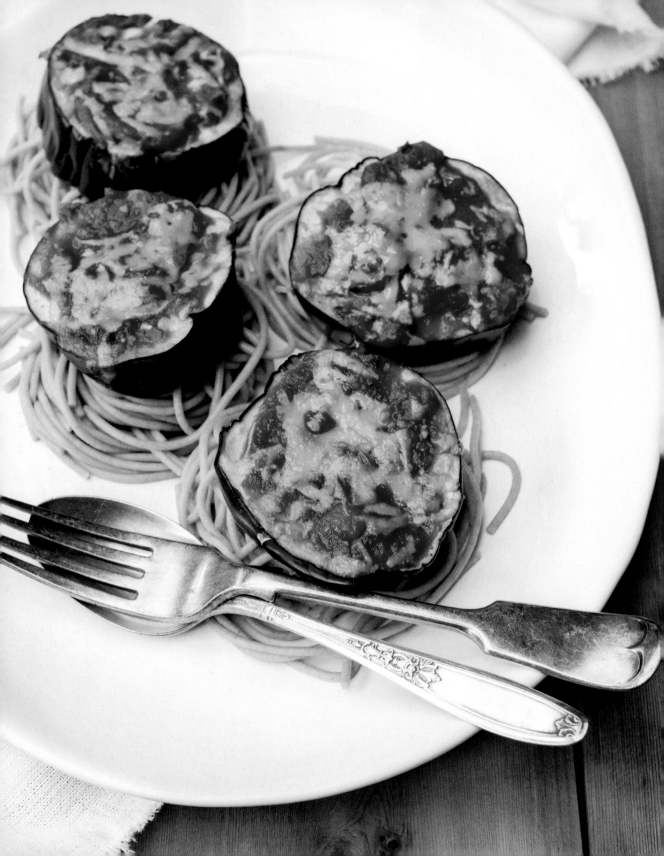

EASY EGGPLANT MARINARA

2 SERVINGS // 20 MINUTES

Plenty of vegetables can be cooked in the microwave. I've found that such shortcuts are a good way to fit a wider variety of vegetables into your diet. If you are counting carbs in hopes of getting closer to your racing weight before the season starts, simply omit the pasta in favor of a healthy spin on minipizzas.

- 4 ounces whole-wheat spaghetti
- 2 teaspoons extra-virgin olive oil
- 1 large eggplant
- 2 tablespoons water
- ½ cup tomato-based pasta sauce
- ½ cup (2 oz.) grated mozzarella cheese
- dried oregano

1 Bring a pot of water to a boil and add spaghetti. Cook 8–10 minutes or as directed on the package. Drain water and return pasta to pot. Toss with olive oil and cover to keep warm.

2 Cut eggplant into 1-inch-thick slices. Place slices on a microwave-safe plate with water. Cover with a damp paper towel and microwave for 3 minutes.

3 Remove paper towel and tilt plate over sink to drain off water. Top each slice with 1 tablespoon sauce and 1 tablespoon cheese.

4 Microwave for 1 minute, then sprinkle with oregano to taste. Serve atop spaghetti.

Per serving: 435 calories, 14 g fat, 63 g total carbohydrate, 13 g dietary fiber, 17 g protein

 TIP

The skin of the eggplant may be bitter or chewy. Simply peel it before cooking if you prefer.

DQS COUNT (per serving) VEGETABLES 1 WHOLE GRAINS 1 DAIRY 1

CAULIFLOWER, WHITE BEAN & CHEDDAR SOUP

2 SERVINGS (2½ CUPS) // 15 MINUTES

You can make this cheesy, high-fiber vegetable soup in minutes. I always keep a bag of frozen cauliflower on hand so I can whip up this soup when I run out of fresh vegetables near the end of the week.

3 cups vegetable broth

1 16-ounce bag _frozen_ cauliflower

¼ cup onion, chopped

2 cloves garlic, minced

1 15-ounce can white beans, drained and rinsed

½ cup (2 oz.) cheddar cheese, grated

salt and pepper

1 Combine broth, cauliflower, onion, garlic, and beans in a pot and bring to a boil. Cook over medium-high heat for 5 minutes, using a wooden spoon to break up the cauliflower into small chunks.

2 Transfer mixture to a blender and puree, or use an immersion blender to puree the soup in the pot. Stir in cheese until melted. Season with salt and pepper to taste.

Per serving: 298 calories, 10 g fat, 40 g total carbohydrate, 14 g dietary fiber, 20 g protein

+ CARBS Add a side of crusty whole-wheat bread for 55 g total carbohydrate.

DQS COUNT (per serving)   VEGETABLES 2 (1 legumes)   DAIRY 1

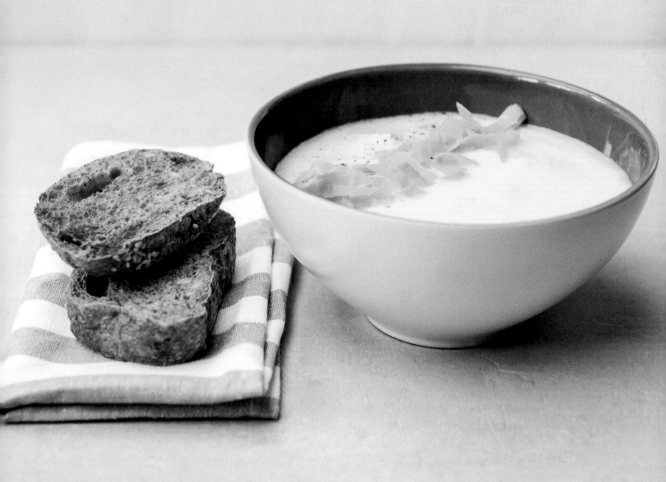

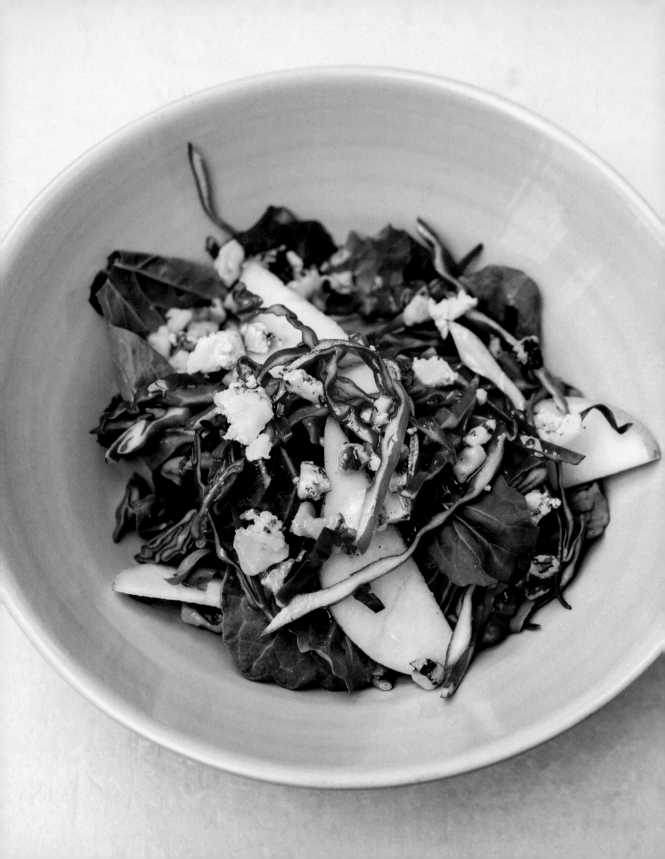

PEAR & BLUE CHEESE SALAD WITH WALNUTS

2 SERVINGS // 10 MINUTES

With sweet, juicy pears, crunchy walnuts, and savory blue cheese, this salad is so full of flavor that you may not even want dressing.

- 6 cups (5 oz.) mixed salad greens, loosely packed
- ½ cup red cabbage, shredded
- 1 pear, thinly sliced
- ½ cup (2 oz.) blue cheese, crumbled
- ¼ cup (1 oz.) walnuts, chopped

1 Arrange salad greens on a plate and top with cabbage, pear, cheese, and walnuts.

2 Serve with dressing of your choice, if desired.

Per serving: 276 calories, 17 g fat, 22 g total carbohydrate, 7 g dietary fiber, 12 g protein

BUYING PREWASHED GREENS

Prewashed bagged lettuce or spinach can make a convenient base for salads, but these products have a short shelf life. To get the freshest greens available, dig through the stock toward the back of the grocery-store shelf, where you are likely to find the bags with expiration dates that are farther out. Don't be shy about grabbing the bag with the latest expiration date.

DQS COUNT (per serving)   FRUITS ½   VEGETABLES 1   NUTS & SEEDS 1   DAIRY 1

ROSEMARY GARLIC CHICKEN

2 SERVINGS // 35 MINUTES

This recipe is the antidote for boring chicken. Bursting with flavor, it's neither complicated nor difficult.

3 cloves garlic, minced

1 tablespoon extra-virgin olive oil

2 teaspoons fresh rosemary leaves, minced

¼ teaspoon salt

⅛ teaspoon black pepper

12 ounces boneless, skinless chicken breast or tenderloins

1 In a small bowl, stir together garlic, olive oil, rosemary, salt, and pepper. Place chicken breasts on a cutting board, and brush both sides with rosemary and garlic mixture.

2 Let chicken rest for 10–20 minutes while preheating indoor or outdoor grill to medium-high heat.

3 When grill is hot, add chicken and cook for 4 minutes on each side or until just cooked through.

Per serving: 251 calories, 9 g fat, 1 g total carbohydrate, 0 g dietary fiber, 39 g protein

+ CARBS Add a medium potato for 32 g total carbohydrate (or a large potato for 45 g).

DQS COUNT (per serving)   LEAN MEATS & FISH   1

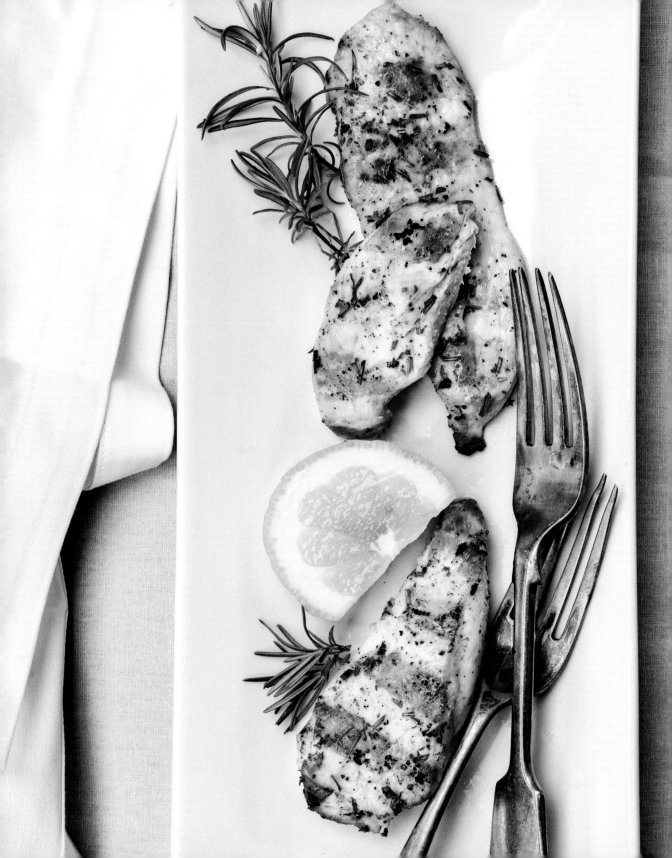

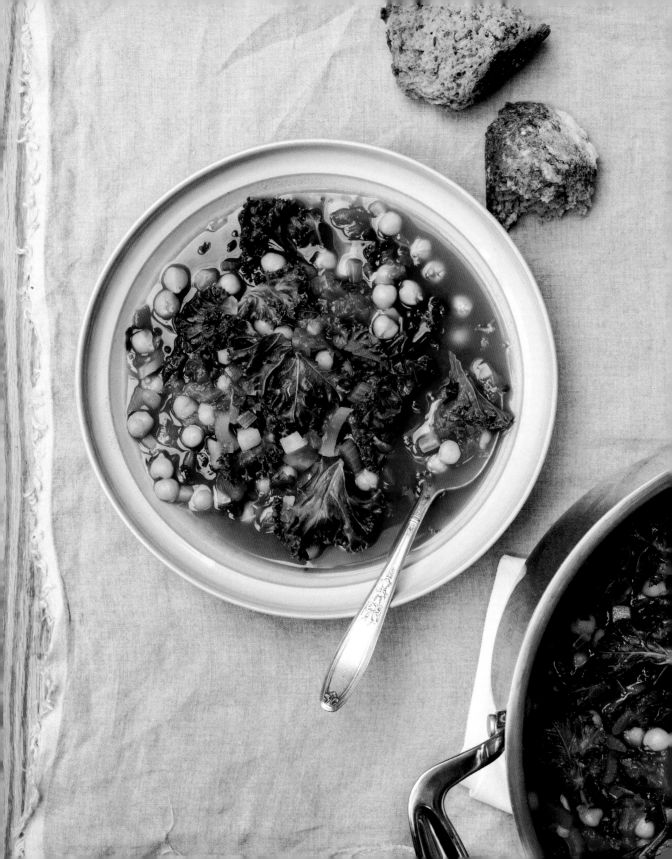

GARDEN MINESTRONE WITH KALE

2 SERVINGS // 50 MINUTES

Chock-full of vegetables and beans, this soup is a hearty, warming meal, packed with nutrition.

- 4 cups vegetable broth
- 1 14½-ounce can diced tomatoes with juice
- 1 15-ounce can garbanzo beans, rinsed and drained
- 1 large carrot, chopped
- 3 ribs celery, chopped
- ½ sweet onion, chopped
- 3 cloves garlic, crushed
- 2 cups baby kale, loosely packed
- 1 handful fresh basil, shredded (optional)
- salt and black pepper

1 Combine all ingredients except kale, salt, and pepper in a large soup pot and bring to a boil. Reduce heat and simmer, covered, for 40 minutes.

2 Add kale and cook for 10 more minutes. Season with fresh basil and salt and pepper to taste.

Per serving: 282 calories, 5 g fat, 55 g total carbohydrate, 17 g dietary fiber, 16 g protein

DQS COUNT (per serving)   VEGETABLES   2½ (1 legumes)

BAKED PORTOBELLO WITH TOMATO

2 SERVINGS // 45 MINUTES

olive-oil cooking spray

2 large portobello
   mushroom caps

1 tablespoon
   balsamic vinegar

1 medium tomato,
   sliced

½ teaspoon dried basil

¼ teaspoon salt

¼ teaspoon
   garlic powder

2 whole-wheat buns
   (optional)

1 Preheat oven to 400 degrees F. Line a baking sheet with parchment paper and coat with cooking spray.

2 Place mushrooms gills-up on baking sheet and mist with cooking spray. Drizzle each cap with ½ tablespoon balsamic vinegar and bake for 20 minutes.

3 Arrange tomato slices on top of mushrooms and sprinkle evenly with basil, salt, and garlic powder. Bake for 15 to 20 minutes more, until tomatoes start to wrinkle.

4 Serve on a whole-wheat bun, if desired, or as a hearty serving of vegetables.

Per serving: 51 calories, 0 g fat, 10 g total carbohydrate, 2 g dietary fiber, 3 g protein

+ CARBS Serve on a whole-wheat bun for 41 g total carbohydrate.

DQS COUNT (per serving)   VEGETABLES 1

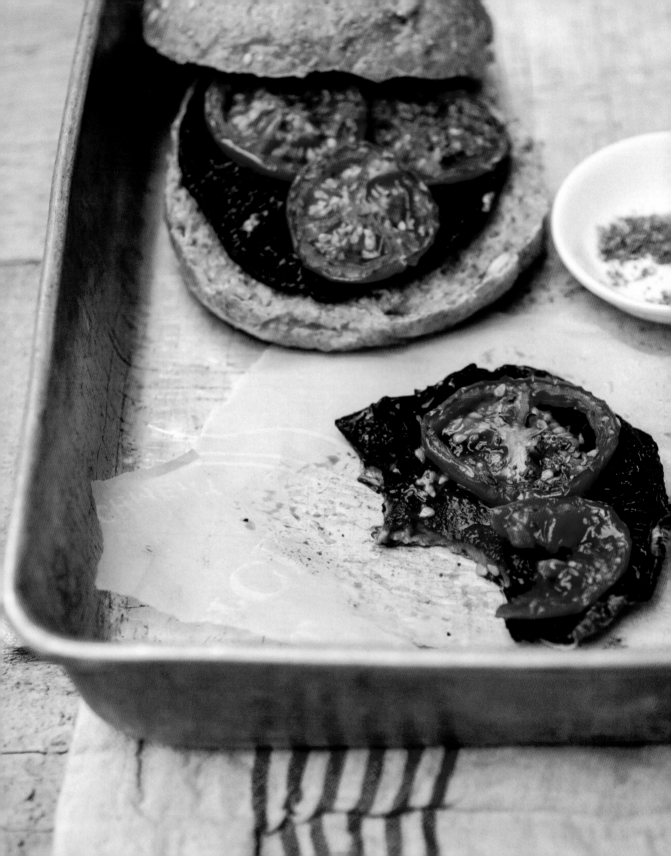

PORK & PEPPER SAUCE OVER ROTINI

4 SERVINGS // 25 MINUTES

1 pound extra-lean
   ground pork

2 cups (8 oz.)
   bell-pepper strips
   (fresh or frozen)

1 24-ounce jar
   marinara sauce

¼ teaspoon
   red pepper flakes

8 ounces whole-wheat
   rotini

1 In a large saucepan, cook pork over medium heat until no
pink remains, using a wooden spoon to break up the meat
as it cooks. Drain fat, if any.

2 Add bell-pepper strips, marinara sauce, and red pepper
flakes to pan. Bring to a boil, then reduce heat and
simmer for 10 minutes, stirring every few minutes. Add more
red pepper flakes, if desired, to achieve desired heat.

3 Bring a large pot of water to a boil and cook pasta for
8–10 minutes or as directed on the package. Drain pasta
and serve topped with sauce.

Per serving: 427 calories, 9 g fat, 56 g total carbohydrate, 10 g dietary fiber,
34 g protein

DQS COUNT (per serving)   VEGETABLES 1   WHOLE GRAINS 1   LEAN MEATS & FISH 1

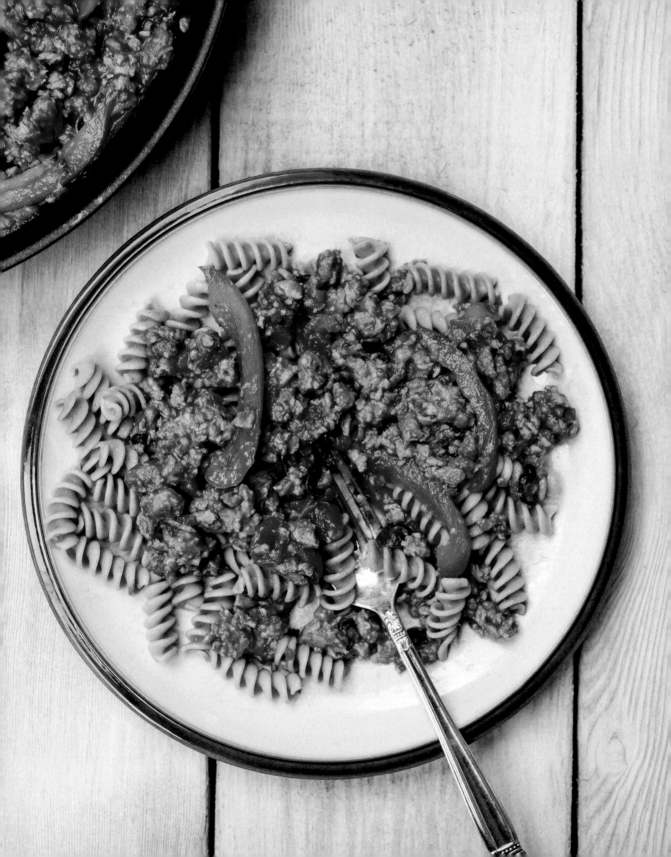

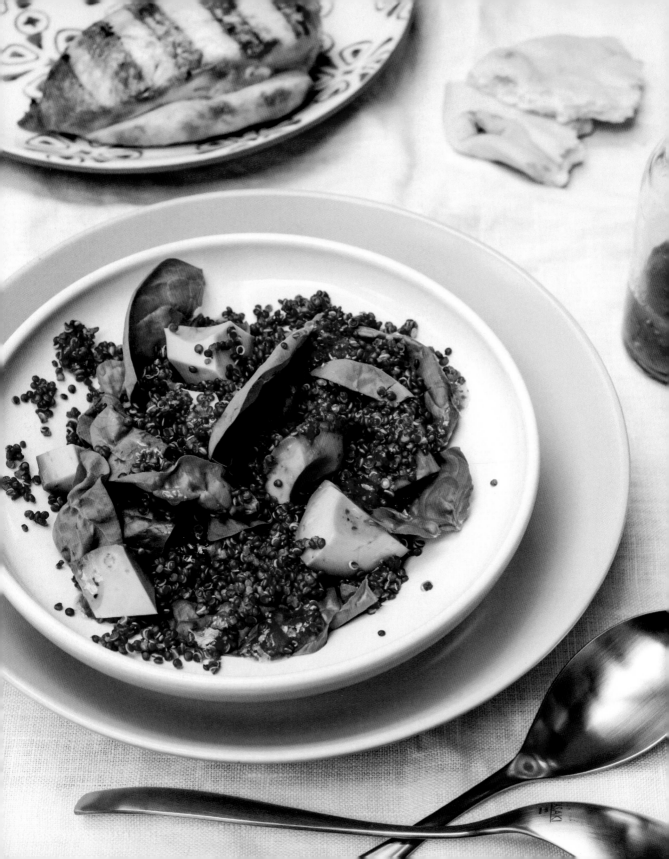

SPINACH SALAD WITH RED QUINOA

2 SERVINGS // 5 MINUTES

- 3 cups fresh baby spinach, loosely packed
- ½ avocado, cubed
- 1 cup *cooked* red quinoa
- ¼ cup sun-dried tomato vinaigrette (or similar dressing)
- 1½ cups *cooked* chicken breast, chopped (optional)

1 In a large bowl, toss together spinach, avocado, cooked quinoa, and vinaigrette to coat evenly.

2 Transfer to a plate and serve with cooked chicken, if desired.

Per serving (without chicken): 247 calories, 13 g fat, 25 g total carbohydrate, 5 g dietary fiber, 6 g protein

Use rotisserie chicken if you don't have cooked chicken breast on hand.

DQS COUNT (per serving)   VEGETABLES   1   WHOLE GRAINS   1

GREEK TORTILLA PIZZA

1 SERVING // 15 MINUTES

1 whole-grain or sprouted-grain tortilla or wrap

½ cup prepared pizza sauce

¼ cup mushrooms, sliced

¼ cup red bell pepper, sliced

¼ cup onion, sliced

2 tablespoons kalamata olives, sliced

2 tablespoons (1 oz.) feta cheese, crumbled

¼ teaspoon dried oregano (optional)

1 Preheat oven to 400 degrees F. Line a baking sheet with foil or parchment paper.

2 Place tortilla on baking sheet and evenly spread with pizza sauce. Top with mushrooms, peppers, onion, olives, and feta. Bake for 10 minutes.

3 Sprinkle with oregano, if desired, before serving. Cut into slices.

Per serving: 277 calories, 15 g fat, 29 g total carbohydrate, 11 g dietary fiber, 15 g protein

WHAT MAKES A GOOD TORTILLA?

Look at the ingredients list and choose a tortilla with whole-wheat flour or sprouted whole wheat as one of the first ingredients (not wheat flour or enriched wheat flour). Scan the rest of the ingredients and make sure they don't include partially hydrogenated oil of any kind. Some of our favorite products are Ezekiel 4:9 Sprouted Whole Grain Tortillas, Flatout whole-grain flatbreads, and Alvarado St. Bakery sprouted-wheat tortillas. La Tortilla Factory white whole-wheat SoftWraps are also a good choice. Sprouted-grain tortillas may be found in the freezer section; the others are usually shelved in a tortilla section or Latin foods aisle.

DQS COUNT (per serving)   VEGETABLES 1   WHOLE GRAINS 1   DAIRY 1

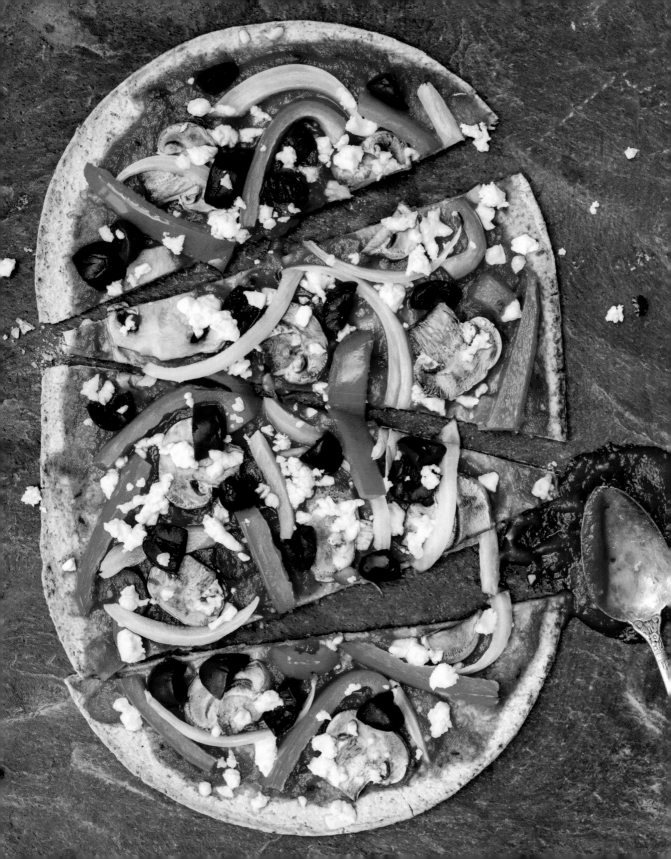

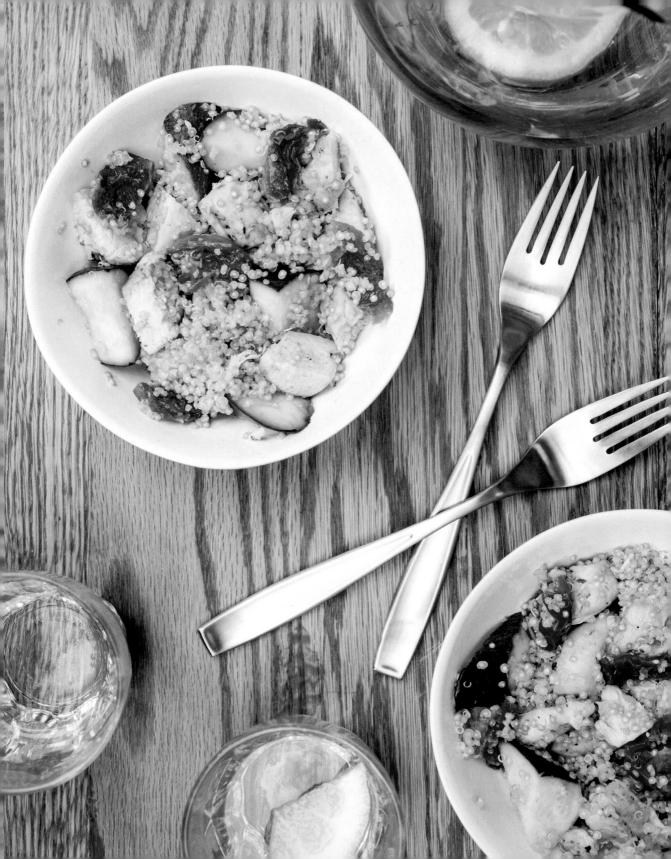

ONE-POT QUINOA, CHICKEN & VEGGIES

4 SERVINGS // 25 MINUTES

Sometimes a complicated meal just isn't going to happen. This is one of my common postworkout meals, a perfect fit for those times when I want some high-quality carbohydrates and protein without a lot of fuss. If you have leftovers, it also makes a great lunch.

2½ cups water

1 cup quinoa, rinsed and drained

2 teaspoons organic chicken or vegetable bouillon

2 cloves garlic, crushed

2½ cups *cooked* chicken breast or rotisserie chicken, chopped

2 zucchini, chopped

½ cup sun-dried tomatoes, coarsely chopped

½ teaspoon dried basil

1 Bring water to a boil in a medium saucepan over high heat. Add quinoa, bouillon, and garlic and return to a boil.

2 Cover, reduce heat to low, and set timer for 20 minutes. After 10 minutes have gone by, stir in chicken, zucchini, sun-dried tomatoes, and basil and cover again.

3 With 2 minutes remaining, remove lid and stir again. Leave pot uncovered to allow any remaining water to evaporate. Scoop into bowls and enjoy.

Per serving: 351 calories, 7 g fat, 39 g total carbohydrate, 5 g dietary fiber, 35 g protein

DQS COUNT (per serving)   VEGETABLES 1   WHOLE GRAINS 1   LEAN MEATS & FISH 1

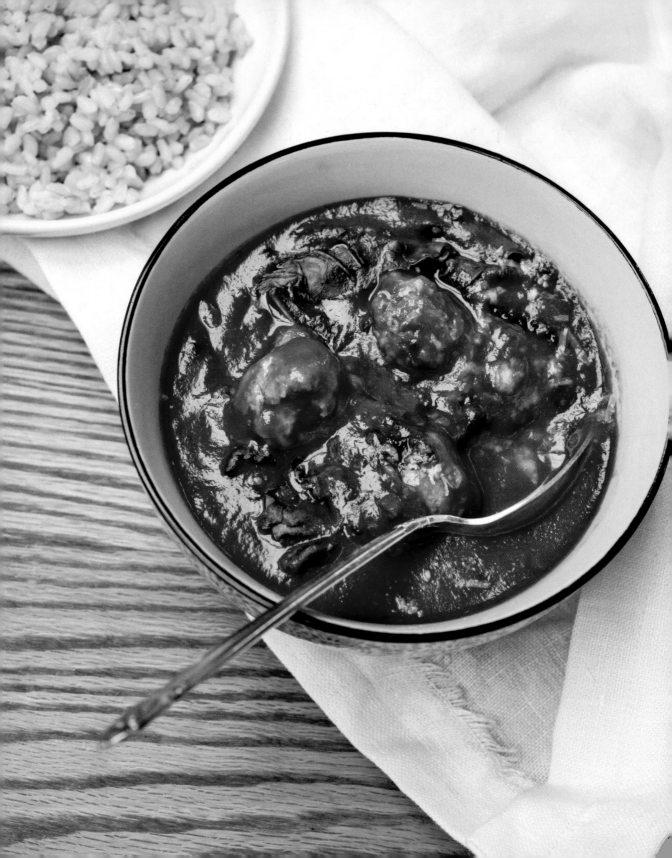

PORTOBELLO & CHICKEN SAUSAGE BOWL

2 SERVINGS // 10 MINUTES

- 2 portobello mushroom caps, sliced
- 2 links (6 oz.) lean chicken sausage, coarsely chopped
- 1 cup water
- 1 8-ounce can tomato sauce
- 2 cups fresh baby spinach, loosely packed
- ¼ cup (¾ oz.) Parmesan cheese, grated

1 Place portobello mushrooms and chicken sausage in a small saucepan with water. Cook over medium-high heat until mushrooms are soft and liquid is reduced, 4–5 minutes.

2 Reduce heat to low and stir in tomato sauce and spinach. Cook, stirring, until mixture begins to simmer and spinach turns bright green and begins to wilt.

3 Remove from heat, divide into two bowls, and stir in Parmesan cheese.

Per serving: 258 calories, 12 g fat, 16 g total carbohydrate, 4 g dietary fiber, 24 g protein

+ CARBS Serve with 1 cup **Basic Brown Rice** (p. 120) for 59 g total carbohydrate.

DQS COUNT (per serving) VEGETABLES 1 LEAN MEATS & FISH 1 DAIRY ½

BEEF & BUTTERNUT SQUASH HASH

2 SERVINGS // 20 MINUTES

This recipe is a great weeknight meal to throw together from a few ingredients. Nutritious, filling, and—since it requires only one pan—easy to clean up!

½ cup water

2 cups _frozen_ butternut squash cubes

8 ounces London broil (top round beef), cubed

2 medium (5 oz. each) zucchini, chopped

2 cups _frozen_ cut leaf spinach thawed, moisture squuzed out

½ teaspoon each salt, cayenne pepper, and cinnamon

1 In a large frying pan bring water to a boil over high heat. Add butternut squash when the water starts to boil. Cook for 5 minutes without stirring. Tilt pan over sink to drain any remaining water.

2 Return pan to heat and add beef, zucchini, spinach, salt, cayenne, and cinnamon. Cook, stirring, until beef is cooked through.

Per serving: 293 calories, 9 g fat, 20 g total carbohydrate, 5 g dietary fiber, 29 g protein

 TIP

Prepare the beef and zucchini chunks to be approximately the same size as the butternut squash cubes so the hash will cook evenly.

DQS COUNT (per serving) VEGETABLES 2 LEAN MEATS & FISH 1

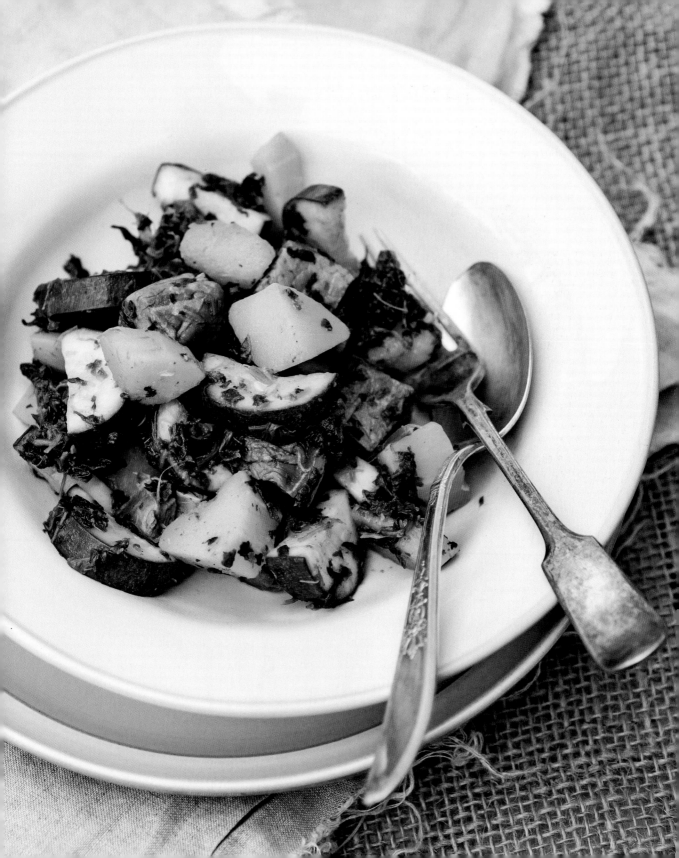

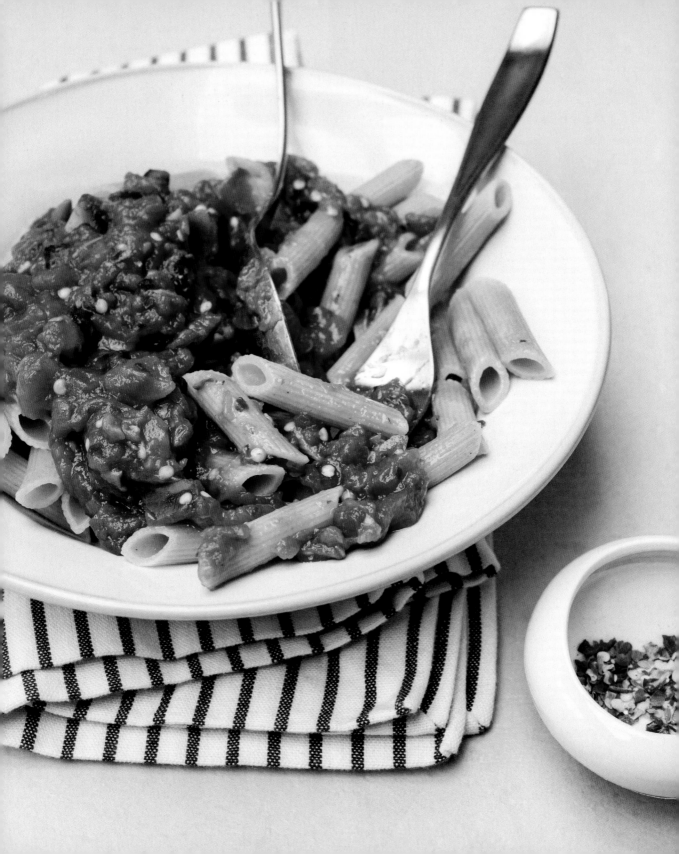

EGGPLANT PRIMAVERA SAUCE

6 SERVINGS (1 CUP) // 15 MINUTES PLUS 6 HOURS IN SLOW COOKER

This slow-cooker recipe takes minimal effort and gives you a big batch of thick, chunky, vegetable-packed sauce. It's great with spaghetti squash or pasta or spooned over chicken.

1 eggplant
(peeled if desired)

8 ounces portobello
mushrooms or
white mushrooms

1 sweet onion

4 cloves garlic, minced

2 14½-ounce cans diced
tomatoes with liquid

1 cup (11 oz.) roasted
red peppers from a jar,
chopped

salt and black pepper

red pepper flakes
(optional)

1 Chop vegetables finely and place in slow cooker. Add canned tomatoes with liquid and roasted red peppers. Cook for 6 hours on low setting.

2 Stir the sauce and season with salt, pepper, and red pepper flakes, if desired, to taste.

Makes 6 cups.

Per serving: 84 calories, 0 g fat, 17 g total carbohydrate, 5 g dietary fiber, 4 g protein

 CARBS Serve with 1 cup whole-wheat pasta for 70 g total carbohydrate.

DQS COUNT (per serving)   VEGETABLES 2

RECIPES FOR

THE ATHLETE WITH SOME COOKING EXPERIENCE

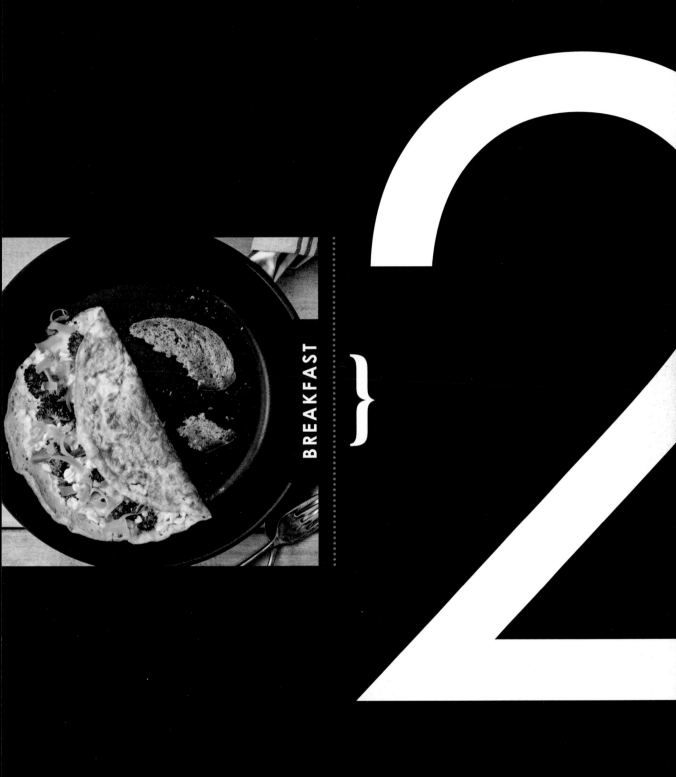

BREAKFAST

}

2

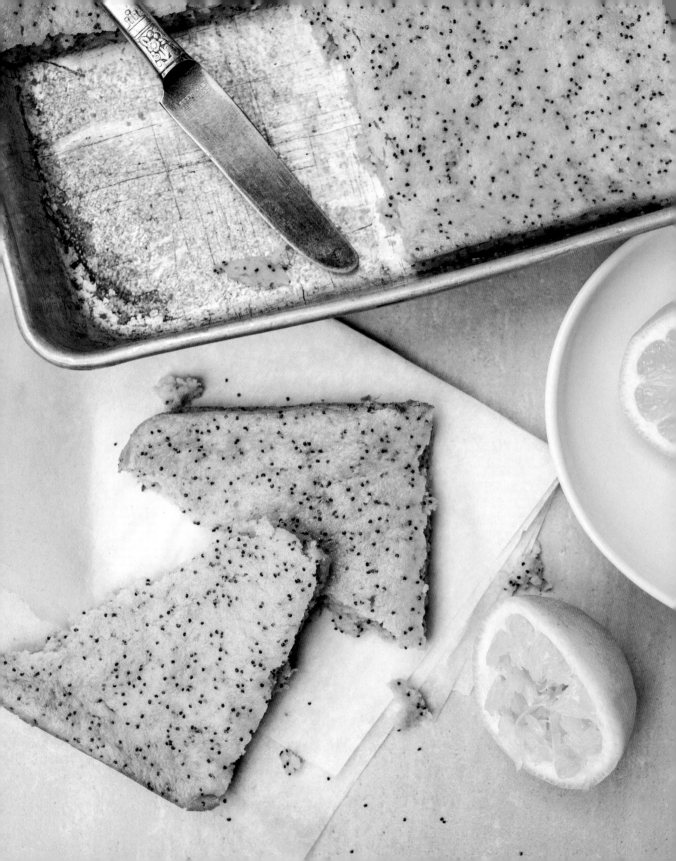

LEMON-POPPY PROTEIN BARS

12 SERVINGS // 40 MINUTES

These light, flavorful bars use white whole-wheat flour, which contains all the nutrition of regular whole-grain flour but has a lighter color and less pronounced flavor that complements this recipe beautifully. If you can't locate white whole-wheat flour, use normal whole-wheat flour.

cooking spray

1⅓ cups white
whole-wheat flour

2 servings (⅔ c.) vanilla
whey protein powder

⅔ cup sugar

2 tablespoons
poppy seeds

2 teaspoons
baking powder

½ teaspoon baking soda

½ teaspoon salt

2 teaspoons lemon zest

1½ cups (12 oz.) nonfat
plain Greek yogurt
(or low-fat or whole)

¾ cup unsweetened
applesauce

1 tablespoon canola oil

2½ teaspoons
lemon extract

2 eggs

1 Preheat oven to 325 degrees F. Coat a 9 × 13-inch pan thoroughly with cooking spray.

2 In a large mixing bowl, combine dry ingredients: flour, whey protein, sugar, poppy seeds, baking powder, baking soda, salt, and zest. Stir to mix.

3 In a separate large mixing bowl, stir together remaining ingredients: yogurt, applesauce, canola oil, lemon extract, and eggs. Add dry ingredients to wet ingredients, and stir just until uniformly moistened. Pour batter into pan.

4 Bake for 25 minutes or until toothpick inserted in center comes out clean. Cool completely before slicing.

Per serving: 145 calories, 3 g fat, 22 g total carbohydrate, 1 g dietary fiber, 8 g protein

If you prefer, these can be baked as 12 standard-sized muffins or 6 jumbo muffins instead of bars. Bake muffins until tops are set (dry to the touch), about 20 minutes.

DQS COUNT (per serving)   WHOLE GRAINS   1

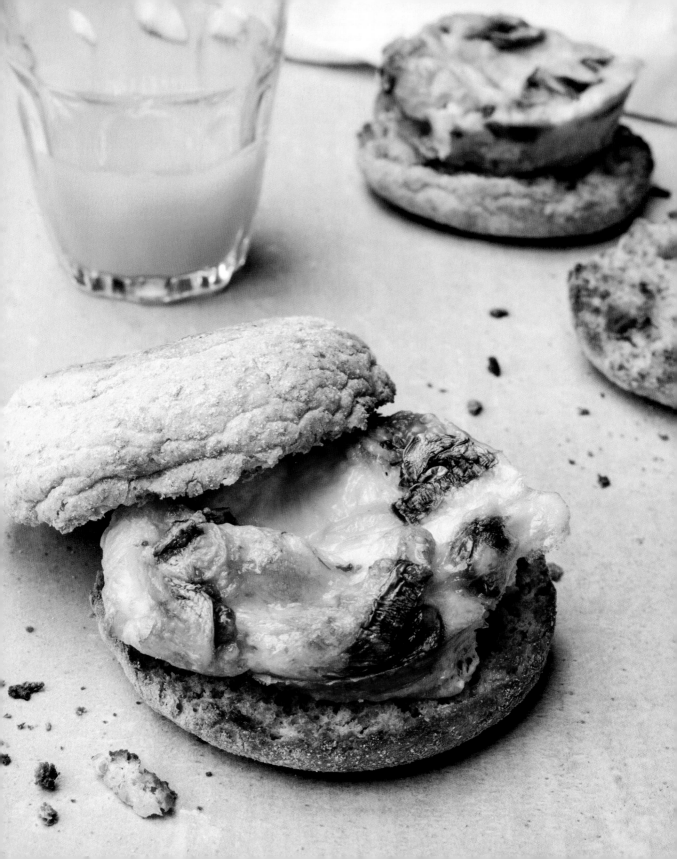

MUSHROOM & PEPPER-JACK EGG MUFFINS

6 SERVINGS (2 MUFFINS) // 35 MINUTES

These little bites are perfect for an instant high-protein breakfast or anytime snack. They are equally tasty hot or cold. Many of my clients pack two of these and an Apple-Bran Muffin (see page 97) for a portable workday breakfast. Try using different types of cheese to vary the flavor.

cooking spray

3 eggs

1½ cups egg whites or egg substitute

6 mushrooms

¾ cup (3 oz.) pepper-jack cheese, grated or chopped

whole-wheat English muffins (optional)

1 Preheat oven to 350 degrees F. Spray a standard 12-muffin tin with cooking spray.

2 In a large bowl, beat together eggs and egg whites, and divide among muffin wells. Chop mushrooms, and divide among muffin wells. (They'll float.)

3 Sprinkle cheese into the egg-mushroom mixture in the muffin wells. (It'll sink.) Bake for 25 minutes, or until toothpick inserted in center comes out clean. Cool for 5–10 minutes before removing from pan.

Store leftovers in refrigerator for up to 5 days.

Per serving: 129 calories, 7 g fat, 1 g total carbohydrate, 1 g dietary fiber, 14 g protein

+ CARBS Make an egg sandwich with a whole-wheat English muffin for 24 g total carbohydrate.

DQS COUNT (per serving)   LEAN MEATS & FISH 1

APPLE-BRAN MUFFINS

12 SERVINGS // 35 MINUTES

cooking spray

1 cup whole-wheat flour

1 cup wheat bran

2 apples (3 c.),
  finely chopped

1 tablespoon
  baking powder

½ teaspoon baking soda

¼ teaspoon salt

½ cup unsweetened
  applesauce

¼ cup skim milk

¼ cup (2) egg whites

¼ cup molasses

2 tablespoons
  extra-virgin olive oil

1 Preheat oven to 350 degrees F. Coat a muffin tin thoroughly with cooking spray.

2 In a large mixing bowl, combine dry ingredients: flour, bran, apples, baking powder, baking soda, and salt. Stir to mix.

3 In a separate large mixing bowl, stir together wet ingredients: applesauce, milk, egg whites, molasses, and oil. Add dry ingredients to wet ingredients, and stir just until uniformly moistened. Spoon batter into 10 muffin wells.

4 Bake for 18–20 minutes or until tops are set to the touch. Allow to cool completely before removing from tin.

Per serving: 108 calories, 3 g fat, 21 g total carbohydrate, 4 g dietary fiber, 3 g protein

DQS COUNT (per serving) WHOLE GRAINS 1

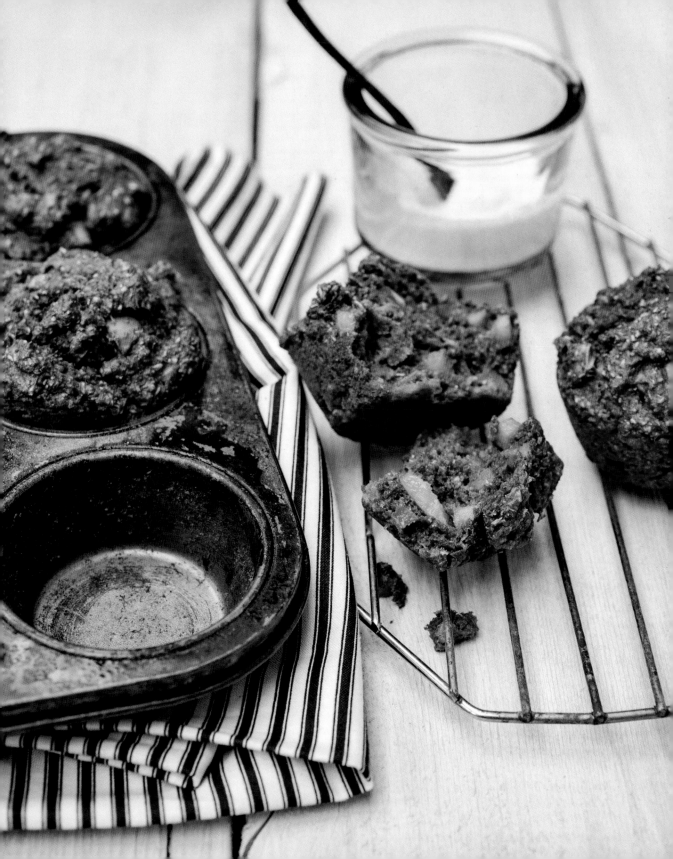

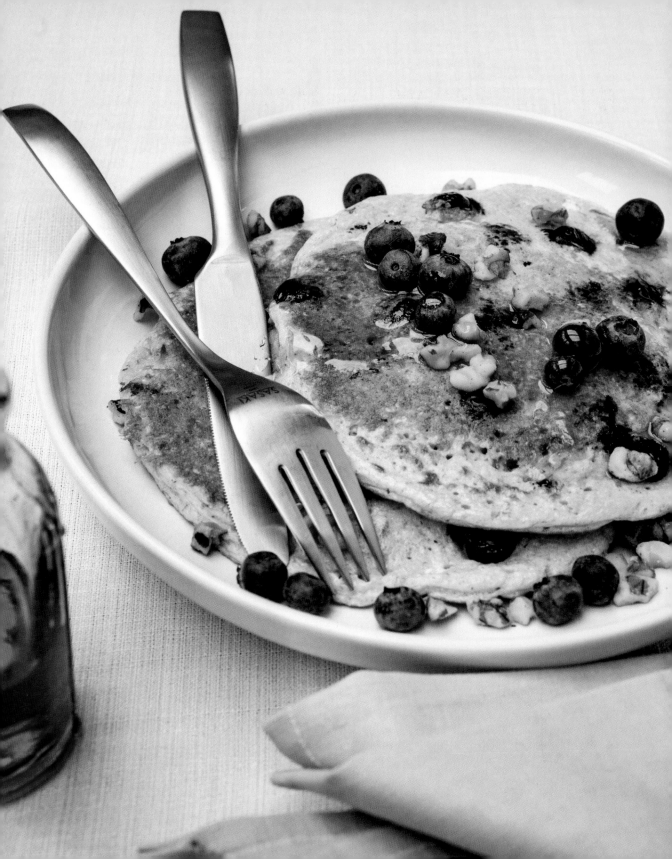

BLUEBERRY-WALNUT PANCAKES

2 SERVINGS (2 PANCAKES) // 15 MINUTES

Blueberries rank high in antioxidants. Add hearty oatmeal and omega-3–rich walnuts, and these pancakes are a deliciously healthy way to start your day.

1 cup oatmeal (old-fashioned or quick oats, not instant)

1 cup egg whites

½ cup 1% cottage cheese

½ tablespoon baking powder

2 tablespoons (½ oz.) walnuts, finely chopped

cooking spray

1 cup blueberries

¼ cup maple syrup (optional)

1 In a blender, combine oatmeal, egg whites, and cottage cheese and process until smooth. Add baking powder and process briefly, just enough to mix it in. Stir in walnuts by hand.

2 Coat a medium nonstick pan with cooking spray and heat over low flame. Pour ½ cup pancake batter into pan. Gently press in several blueberries as the pancake begins to cook.

3 When pancake is golden underneath (use spatula to peek), flip and cook for a few minutes on the other side. Transfer cooked pancake to a plate, and repeat with remaining batter and blueberries. Serve with maple syrup, if desired.

Makes 4 pancakes.

Per serving: 330 calories, 8 g fat, 39 g total carbohydrate, 7 g dietary fiber, 21 g protein

Blueberries are at their peak in the summer, but frozen berries can be found year-round and are an acceptable substitute.

DQS COUNT (per serving)   FRUITS ½   WHOLE GRAINS 1   NUTS & SEEDS ½

PUMPKIN & MAPLE-NUT OATMEAL

2 SERVINGS // 15 MINUTES

For a well-rounded breakfast, have a hard-boiled egg or two with this bowl of oatmeal. You'll be set with high-fiber carbohydrate, healthy fat, and protein to keep you full for hours.

3 cups water

¾ cup canned pumpkin

½ teaspoon salt

1½ cup rolled oats
(also called
old-fashioned oats)

1 tablespoon
pumpkin-pie spice

2 tablespoons (½ oz.)
pecans, chopped

2 tablespoons
maple syrup

1 Combine water, pumpkin, and salt in a small saucepan and bring to a boil.

2 Add oats and pumpkin-pie spice. When mixture starts to bubble again, turn heat down to low. Cook, stirring occasionally, until oats are cooked and cereal has thickened, about 8 minutes.

3 Split between two bowls and top with pecans and maple syrup.

Per serving: 362 calories, 9 g fat, 63 g total carbohydrate, 11 g dietary fiber, 10 g protein

Freeze leftover pumpkin in ice-cube trays; each cube is about 1 ounce.

DQS COUNT (per serving) VEGETABLES ½ WHOLE GRAINS 1 NUTS & SEEDS ½

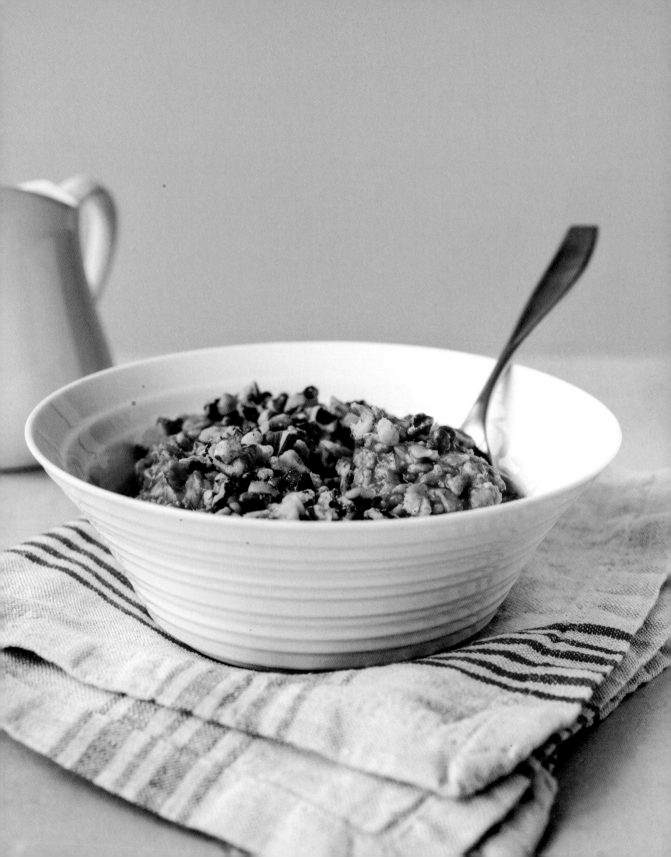

COCONUT-BANANA PROTEIN BARS

4 SERVINGS // 25 MINUTES

cooking spray

1 cup egg whites

1 banana, mashed

1 tablespoon coconut oil, melted

1½ cups quick oats

½ cup sugar

½ teaspoon baking powder

¼ teaspoon salt

1 serving (⅓ c.) vanilla whey protein powder

1 tablespoon coconut flakes (optional)

1 Preheat oven to 375 degrees F. Use cooking spray to lightly grease a 9-inch round cast-iron skillet (or cake pan).

2 In a large bowl, mix together egg whites, mashed banana, and coconut oil.

3 In a second bowl, mix together oats, sugar, baking powder, salt, and whey protein. Add wet ingredients to dry ingredients and stir until uniform. Spread in prepared pan and top with coconut flakes, if desired. Bake for 14 minutes.

4 Cool and cut into generous servings. Wrap in plastic and refrigerate.

Per serving: 308 calories, 6 g fat, 51 g total carbohydrate, 4 g dietary fiber, 17 g protein

For more coconut flavor, add ½ teaspoon coconut extract.

DIVIDE AND CONQUER

It's all too easy to eat bigger portions when you make a large batch of something. For portion control, predivide bars or single servings of food and package them individually in plastic wrap or small containers. This makes them handy to grab and go if you're in a rush; plus they are out of sight in the freezer and less likely to tempt you to eat them when you aren't actually hungry.

DQS COUNT (per serving)   WHOLE GRAINS 1   LEAN MEATS & FISH 1

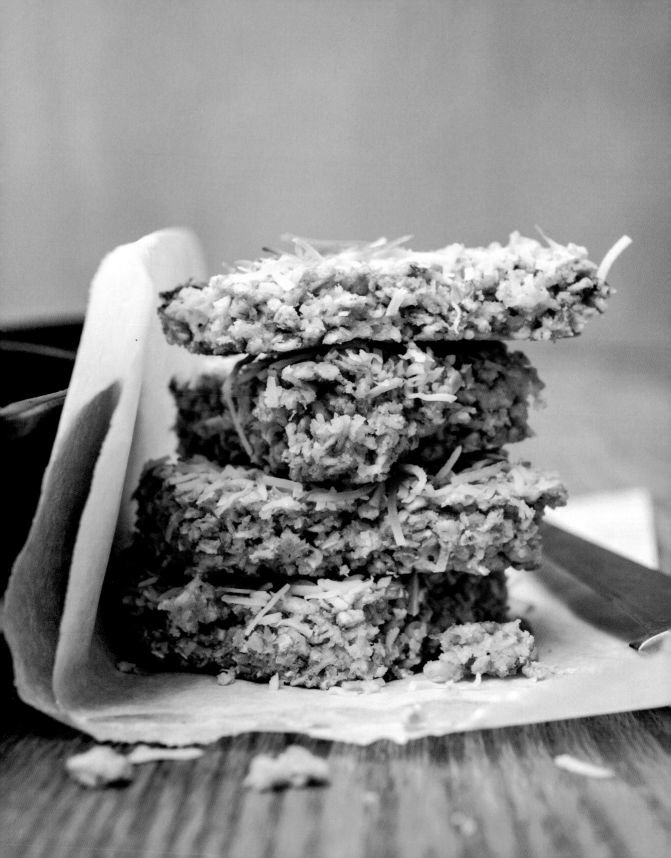

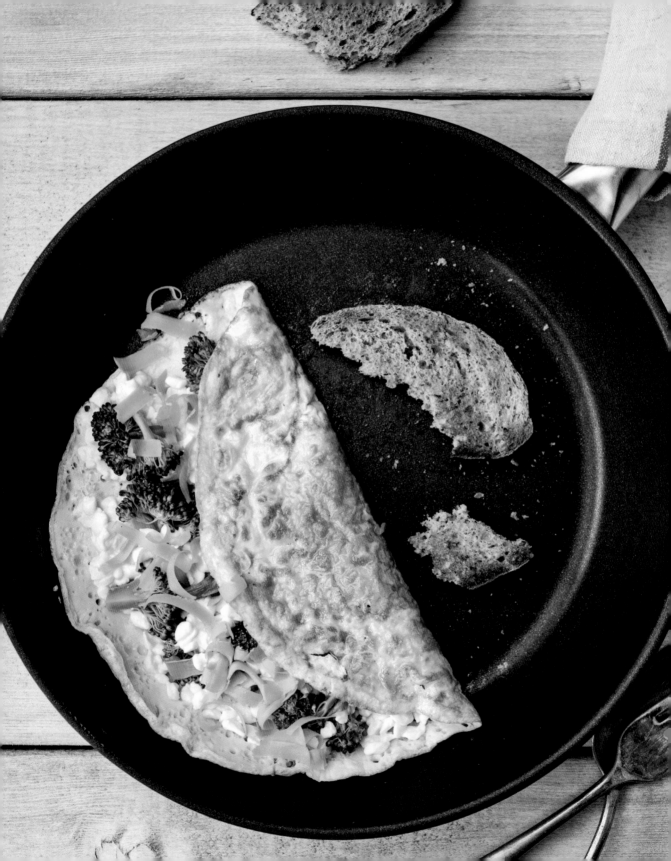

BROCCOLI-CHEESE OMELET

1 SERVING // 15 MINUTES

½ cup broccoli, chopped

¼ cup 1% cottage cheese

¼ cup (1 oz.) cheddar cheese, grated

cooking spray

1 egg

½ cup (4) egg whites

1 Place broccoli in microwave-safe bowl and cook 60 seconds to soften. Add cottage cheese and cheddar cheese to the broccoli and stir to combine.

2 Coat a medium nonstick skillet with cooking spray and heat over medium-low heat. Lightly beat egg and egg whites; pour into pan. Distribute broccoli-and-cheese mixture evenly over eggs.

3 Cook until eggs are solid and cheeses are melted, then gently fold omelet in half and slide onto plate.

Per serving: 288 calories, 14 g fat, 6 g total carbohydrate, 1 g dietary fiber, 32 g protein

+ CARBS Add 2 slices of toasted whole-grain bread for 36 g total carbohydrate.

DQS COUNT (per serving) | VEGETABLES ½ | LEAN MEATS & FISH 1 | DAIRY ½

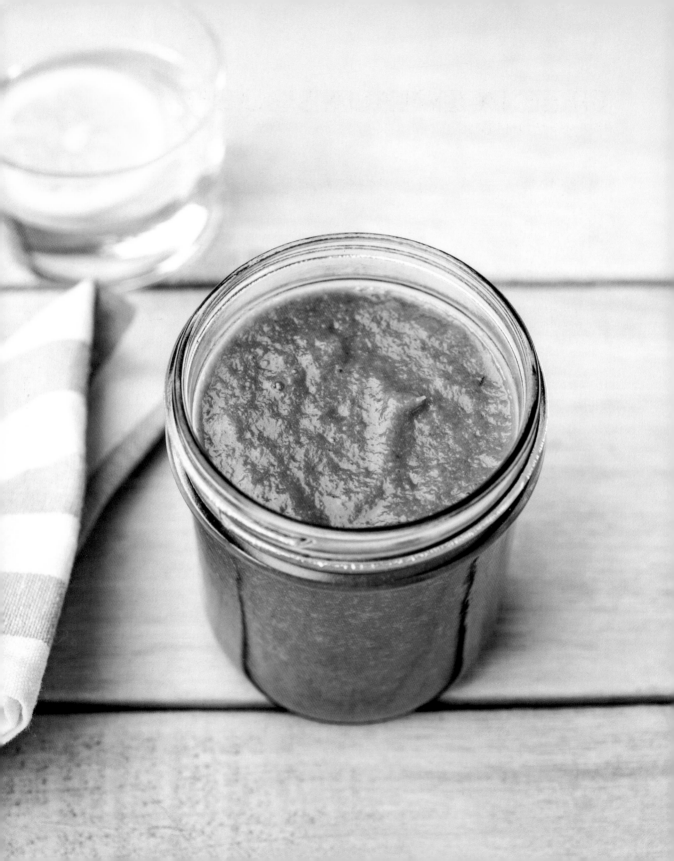

GREENA COLADA SMOOTHIE

1 SERVING // 5 MINUTES

1 14-ounce can crushed pineapple in juice (unsweetened)

¼ cup canned coconut milk

1 cup baby spinach, loosely packed

1 serving protein powder (optional)

1 Blend all ingredients until smooth.

Makes one 16-ounce smoothie.

Per serving: 400 calories, 11 g fat, 66 g carbohydrate, 4 g dietary fiber, 2 g protein

WHY USE PROTEIN POWDER?

Protein powder can be a convenient way to meet your protein needs, whether you are making hot cereal for a preworkout breakfast, blending a recovery smoothie, or baking for postworkout snacks. We recommend buying a whey protein powder that is low in fat and sugar and is free of additional anabolic ingredients (e.g., creatine monohydrate) that are unnecessary for endurance athletes. Look for a basic whey protein powder with 20 or more grams of protein and fewer than 175 calories per serving (typically 30 g). If you have an allergy or intolerance to whey or dairy protein, soy protein is a generally tasty alternative. As for flavors, vanilla is the most versatile and complements all other tastes.

Feel free to omit protein powder from your smoothies. In baked goods, you can simply add the equivalent amount of flour.

DQS COUNT (per serving)   FRUITS 1   VEGETABLES 1

ALMOND & FRUIT GRANOLA

12 SERVINGS (¼ CUP) // 30 MINUTES

3 tablespoons smooth natural almond butter

3 tablespoons honey

¼ teaspoon vanilla extract

¼ teaspoon salt

1 cup rolled oats (also called old-fashioned oats)

⅓ cup (1½ oz.) sliced almonds

¼ cup (1 oz., about 4) dried apricots, chopped

¼ cup (1 oz., about 4) dried figs, chopped

¼ cup raisins

1 Preheat oven to 300 degrees F. Line a baking sheet with parchment paper.

2 In a medium bowl, combine almond butter, honey, vanilla, and salt and stir to mix. Heat in microwave for 20 seconds if almond butter doesn't melt and mix in easily. Add oats and almonds, and gently fold to combine.

3 Scoop mixture onto cookie sheet and spread out; it will form small clumps. Bake for 10 minutes, then turn off the oven and allow to cool completely with the oven door slightly open. Granola will get crunchy as it cools.

4 Mix in dried fruit when granola has cooled. Store granola in a sealed plastic bag.

Makes about 3 cups.

Per serving: 109 calories, 4 g fat, 17 g total carbohydrate, 2 g dietary fiber, 2 g protein

DRIED FRUIT, HOLD THE SUGAR

When buying dried fruit, check the ingredients list for added sweeteners. When possible, choose varieties that are just fruit without sugar, corn syrup, or sucrose listed among the ingredients. Apricots, raisins, dates, figs, and prunes are often sold unsweetened, but blueberries, cranberries, strawberries, papaya, and pineapple usually have added sugar.

DQS COUNT (per serving)   WHOLE GRAINS ½

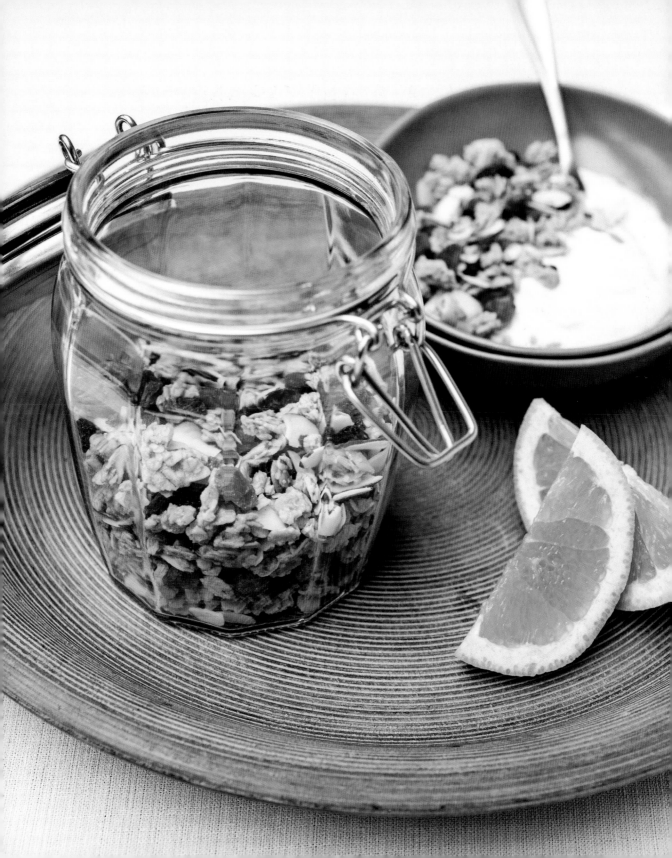

BANANA-PECAN PANCAKES

2 SERVINGS (2 PANCAKES) // 15–20 MINUTES R V

These pancakes are a great make-ahead breakfast. Double the batch, and store pancakes in freezer bags to be reheated in the toaster. They are delicious on their own, but you can top them with syrup or additional sliced banana if you like.

1 cup oats

1 cup egg whites

½ cup 1% cottage cheese

1 banana

1 teaspoon vanilla extract

2 teaspoons baking powder

cooking spray (or ½ tsp. butter)

¼ cup (1 oz.) pecans, chopped

1 Combine oats, egg whites, cottage cheese, banana, and vanilla in a blender and process until completely smooth. Add baking powder and process for just a second or two to mix in.

2 Heat a nonstick skillet over medium heat and coat with cooking spray or butter. Pour in about one-quarter of the batter to make a 7-inch pancake, and sprinkle with 1 tablespoon chopped pecans.

3 Cook until the bottom of the pancake is golden brown, then flip and cook the other side for a few minutes. Repeat with remaining batter and pecans.

Makes 4 large pancakes.

Per serving: 404 calories, 14 g fat, 44 g total carbohydrate, 7 g dietary fiber, 29 g protein

DQS COUNT (per serving)   FRUITS ½   WHOLE GRAINS 1   LEAN MEATS & FISH 1   NUTS & SEEDS 1

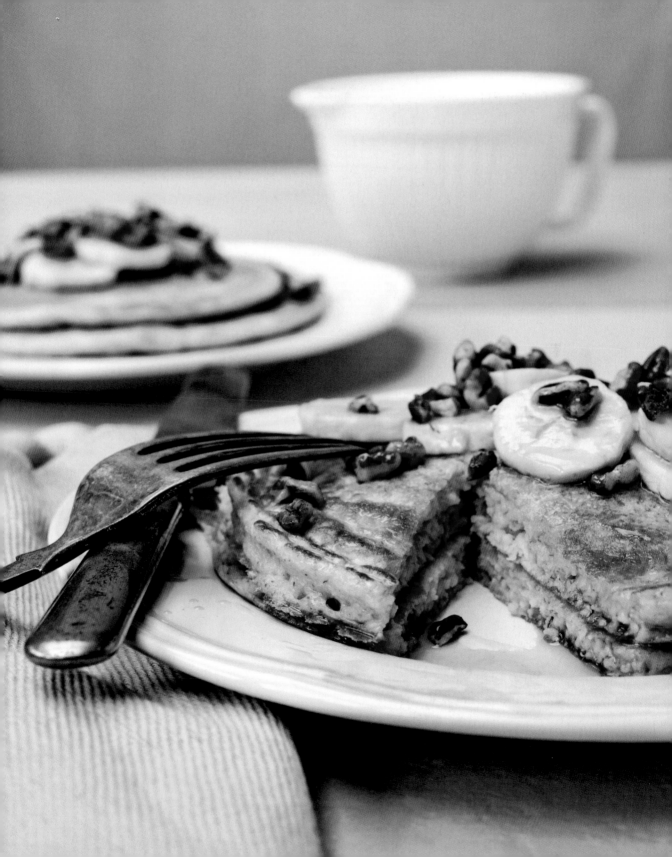

GREENS, EGGS & YAM

2 SERVINGS // 20 MINUTES

Here's a hearty breakfast or brunch for two. You can use Swiss chard or spinach—both are rich in minerals and phytonutrients. Change up the flavor with different cheeses, or omit cheese altogether.

cooking spray

4 cups Swiss chard, chopped and loosely packed

½ medium (4 oz.) sweet potato, grated

½ cup yellow onion, chopped

¼ teaspoon seasoned salt

⅛ teaspoon cayenne pepper (optional)

4 eggs

¼ cup (2 oz.) feta cheese, crumbled

1 Coat a large nonstick skillet with cooking spray and heat over medium heat. When hot, add chard, sweet potato, and onion. Cook, stirring occasionally, until vegetables are tender, about 5 minutes. Sprinkle with seasoned salt and cayenne.

2 Use a spatula to make four wells in the vegetables, and crack an egg into each well. Cover pan and cook until yolks are done to your liking, about 5 minutes.

3 Divide between two plates and sprinkle with crumbled cheese.

Per serving: 253 calories, 12 g fat, 19 g total carbohydrate, 5 g dietary fiber, 19 g protein

DQS COUNT (per serving)   VEGETABLES 1   LEAN MEATS & FISH 1   DAIRY ½

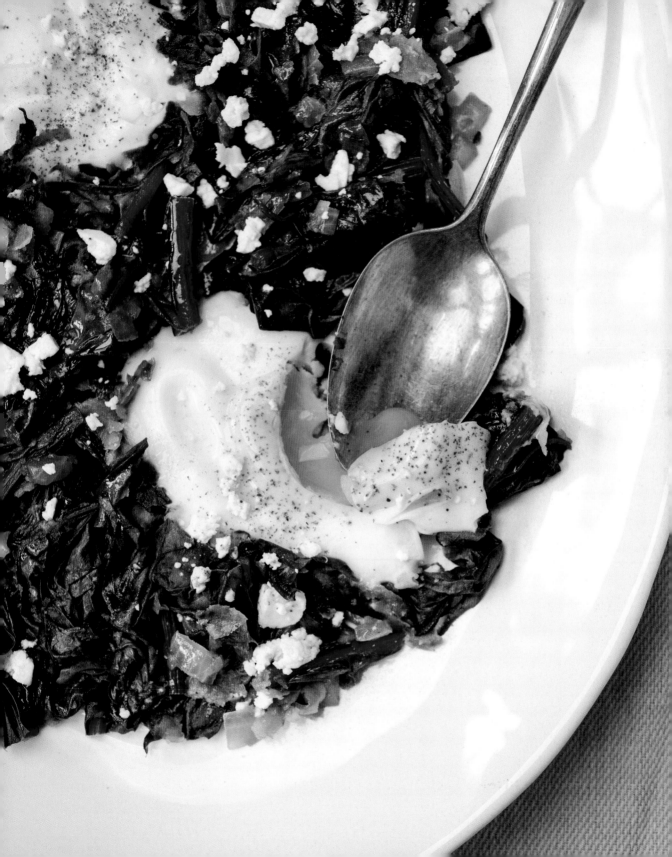

EAT HEALTHY ANYWHERE

Most people—athletes included—eat less healthfully outside the home than they do under their own roofs. But it doesn't have to be that way. Armed with a few basic principles, you can sustain a high-quality diet on road trips, at airports and on airplanes, in sports arenas, on dates at fancy restaurants, and in virtually any other circumstance. Here are our top five rules for eating healthy anywhere.

Don't get trapped. The risk of consuming low-quality meals is greatest when we find ourselves hungry and ready to eat in environments where there aren't a lot of healthy options. Avoiding such traps requires a little forethought. Eat a healthy meal right before you head to the basketball arena, where the "healthiest" foods served may be giant pretzels and nachos. Instead of trying to find the healthiest thing on the menu at Earl's Barbecue Pit, take your date to a different sort of restaurant, where he can get the baby-back ribs he likes and you can choose from many healthier menu items.

> **TIP** *Buy a big salad at the airport to take with you on your flight, where no vegetable will be served.*

Collect solutions. Only a handful of situations will threaten your intentions of eating healthfully away from home. Chances are you've experienced all of these situations before, and you will continue to run into them again and again. You need only solve each of these situations once. After that you can apply the same solution over and over. For example, you may occasionally find yourself having to shop at a convenience store for something to quiet your hunger. There are some reasonably nutritious items to be found. Once you've identified the specific items that work best for you, seek them out whenever you find yourself in the same situation.

> **TIP** *Most convenience stores carry some selection of healthier snacks such as KIND bars, jerky, nuts, and bottled smoothies.*

In a pinch, go small. There will be rare occasions when you will find yourself needing to eat in a situation where there simply are no high-quality foods available. Make the best of these occasions by eating the smallest amount of the healthiest possible available option that will tide you over until you can obtain a high-quality meal somewhere else. When my stomach rumbles at a movie theater, I sometimes buy a bag of peanut M&Ms (at least it has peanuts!) and eat half the bag or less.

Maintain your standards. You wake up in a business hotel room. After dressing, you take the elevator down to the breakfast buffet, where you eye the various offerings and then load your plate with greasy sausage and pastries (things you never eat at home) while thinking, *It's okay, I'm traveling.* If this scenario is familiar, you're not alone. The primary reason people eat less healthfully away from home is that they lower their standards. But instead of acknowledging this slippage, they rationalize their choices with the thought that they are making a rare exception or that it's impossible to eat the same away from home as they do at home.

These "rare exceptions" are never as rare as we like to think, and while it may be next to impossible to eat exactly the same foods on the road that you eat at home, you can still eat just as well. You may be amazed at

what a difference it makes to consciously choose not to lower your diet quality standards when you leave home. Suddenly all kinds of options that you overlooked before become visible.

TIP *Most business-hotel breakfast buffets offer hard-boiled eggs, at least one whole-grain breakfast cereal, fresh fruit, yogurt, and 100 percent fruit juices.*

Play vegetarian. A vegetarian diet isn't necessarily healthier than one that includes high-quality animal foods, but "playing" vegetarian can be an effective way to find and choose healthier foods to eat when you find yourself in an unfamiliar place. On a recent trip to Miami Beach, I used my smart phone to search for vegetarian eateries near my hotel and eventually found Maoz, a fast-service falafel and vegetarian restaurant. I bought a delicious, vegetable-filled whole-wheat pita sandwich and fresh-squeezed fruit juice at Maoz for less than $20 after having passed numerous pizza and burger joints on the walk over there.

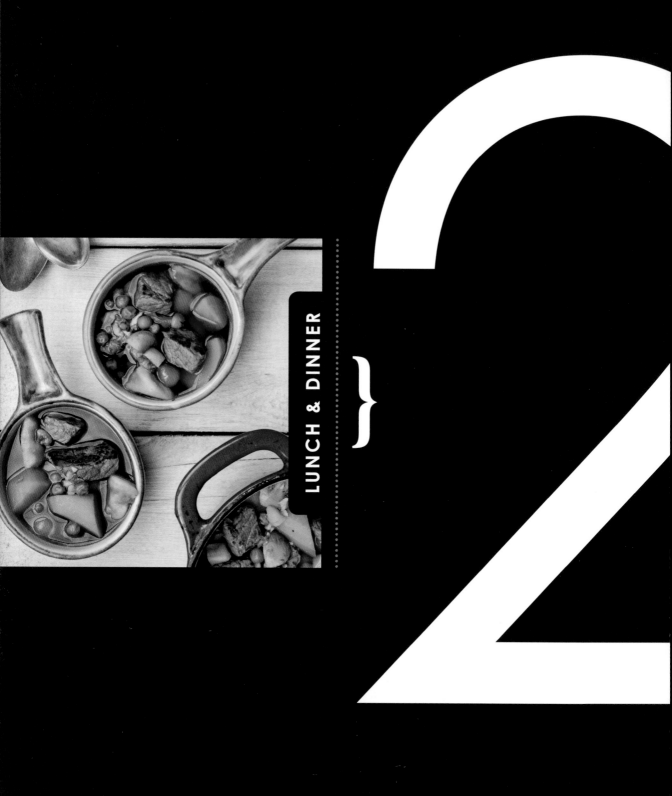

LUNCH & DINNER

2

THE ATHLETE WITH SOME COOKING EXPERIENCE

BROWN RICE
4 WAYS

3 SERVINGS // 50 MINUTES

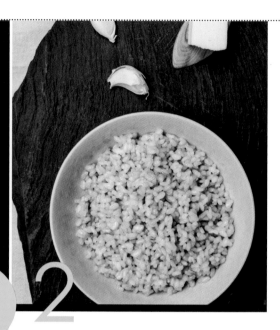

1

BASE FOR NEXT 3 RECIPES

BASIC BROWN RICE

1 cup long-grain brown rice
2½ cups water

Rinse and drain rice. Bring water to a boil and stir in rice. When water returns to a boil, reduce heat to low and cover. Cook for 40–50 minutes, until rice is tender and most liquid has been absorbed.

Turn off heat and leave rice in the covered pot for 5 minutes before fluffing with a fork.

Makes 3 cups cooked rice.

Per serving: 200 calories, 1 g fat, 43 g total carbohydrate, 0 g dietary fiber, 4 g protein

DQS COUNT (per serving)

WHOLE GRAINS	1

2

GARLIC & BUTTER BROWN RICE

3 cups *cooked* brown rice
1 tablespoon butter
1 teaspoon garlic powder
¼ teaspoon salt

Stir butter, garlic powder, and salt into hot cooked rice.

Per serving: 261 calories, 5 g fat, 48 g total carbohydrate, 3 g dietary fiber, 5 g protein

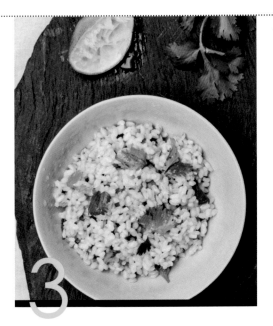

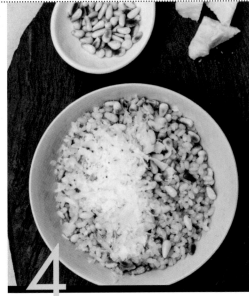

3

CILANTRO-LIME BROWN RICE

  3 cups _cooked_ brown rice

  ½ cup chopped cilantro

  1 tablespoon lime juice

  ¼ teaspoon salt

  ⅛ teaspoon pepper

Stir cilantro, lime juice, salt, and pepper into hot cooked rice.

Per serving: 228 calories, 1 g fat, 48 g total carbohydrate, 3 g dietary fiber, 5 g protein

4

BROWN RICE WITH TOASTED PINE NUTS & PARMESAN ⒽⒸ

  3 cups _cooked_ brown rice

  ¼ cup pine nuts

  ¼ cup Parmesan cheese, coarsely grated

  ¼ teaspoon salt

  ⅛ teaspoon pepper

Place pine nuts in a dry skillet over medium-low heat. Shake every minute or so to roll them around, and remove them from the skillet when fragrant and lightly browned.

Stir toasted pine nuts, Parmesan, salt, and pepper into hot cooked rice.

Per serving: 321 calories, 8 g fat, 51 g total carbohydrate, 3 g dietary fiber, 9 g protein

ARUGULA, BARLEY & BLACKBERRY SALAD

2 SERVINGS // 5 MINUTES

6 cups (5 oz.) baby arugula, loosely packed

1 pint blackberries

1 cup red onion, sliced

1 cup red pepper, sliced into strips

2 cups _cooked_ barley

1 Combine arugula, blackberries, onion, pepper, and cooked barley. Gently toss together and serve.

Per serving: 307 calories, 2 g fat, 70 g total carbohydrate, 17 g dietary fiber, 7 g protein

DQS COUNT (per serving)   FRUITS 1   VEGETABLES 1   WHOLE GRAINS 1

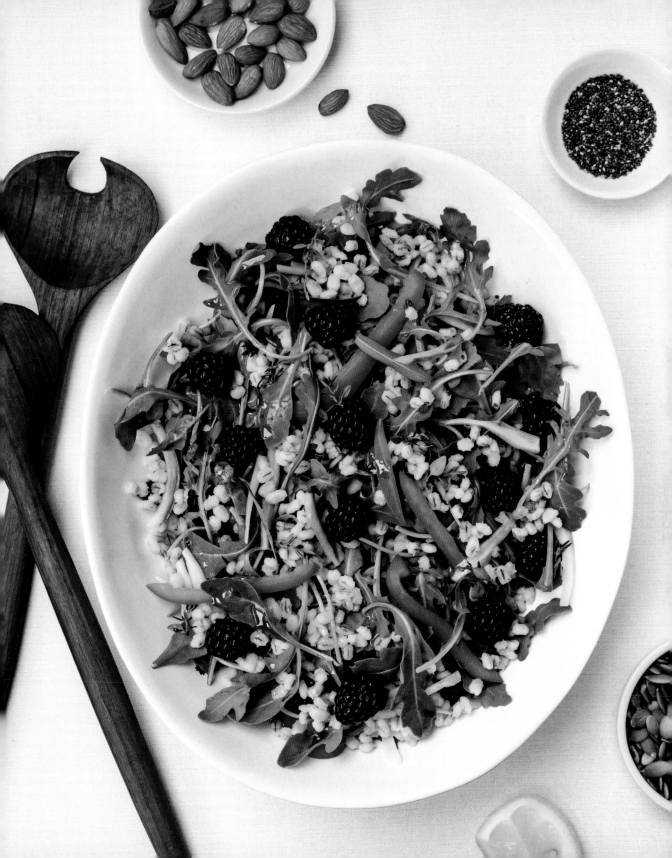

ROASTED RED PEPPER & RED LENTIL SOUP

2 SERVINGS // 30 MINUTES

I've served this soup when entertaining guests, and no one could guess what the two main ingredients were. But they all agreed they loved it! The lentils will actually be a paler color after cooking, but the soup gets a lovely red hue once the peppers are added.

½ cup red lentils

4 cups vegetable broth

2 tablespoons dried onion flakes

2 cloves garlic, quartered

1 cup (11 oz.) roasted red peppers from a jar

sour cream (optional)

1 Combine lentils, broth, onion flakes, and garlic in a small saucepan and bring to a boil over medium-high heat. Reduce heat to low and simmer for 20 minutes.

2 Remove from heat and let cool for 5 minutes.

3 Transfer soup into blender pitcher and add roasted red peppers. Pulse until completely smooth. Season to taste with salt and pepper. Garnish with sour cream, if desired.

Per serving: 226 calories, 0 g fat, 40 g total carbohydrate, 10 g dietary fiber, 14 g protein

DQS COUNT (per serving)   VEGETABLES   1½ (½ legumes)

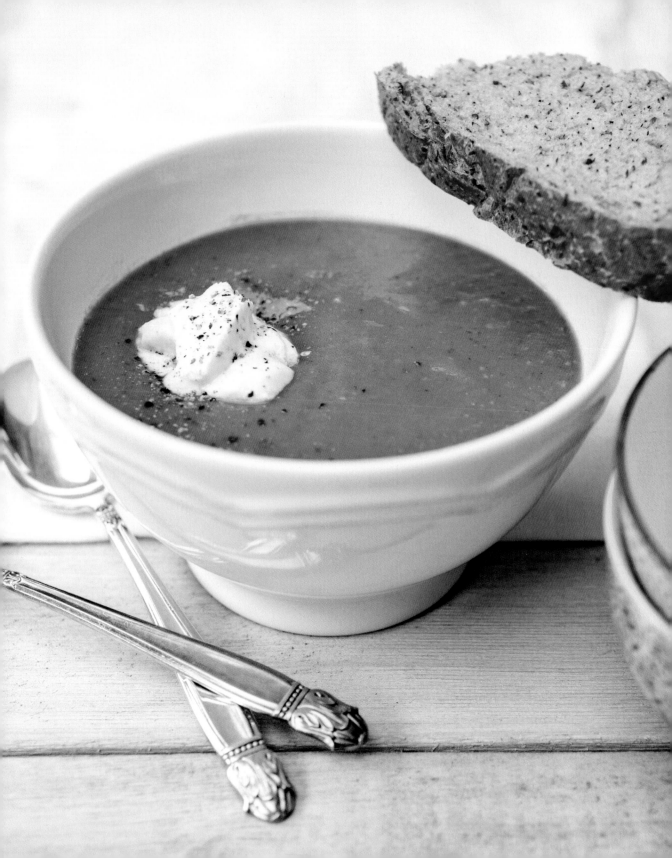

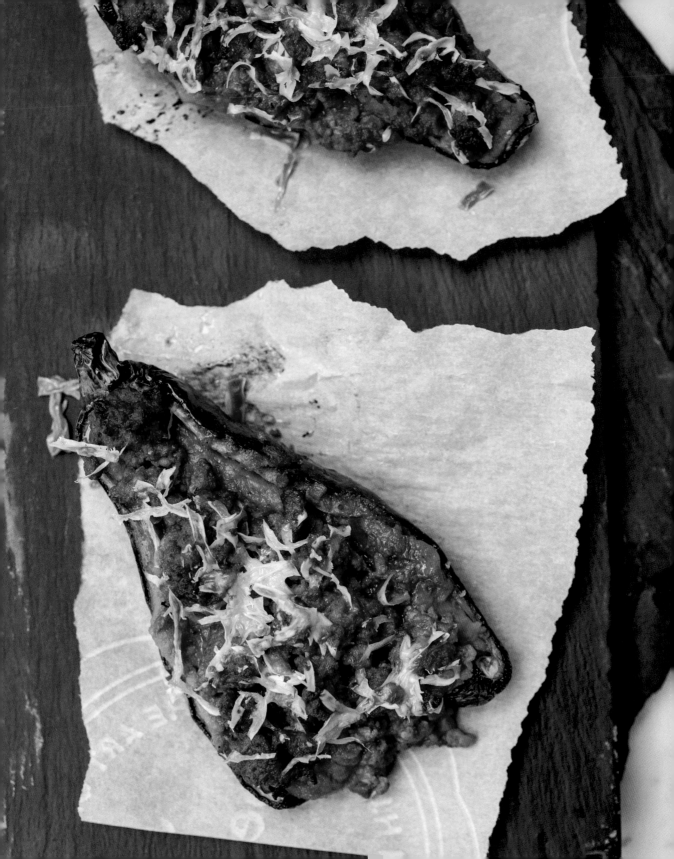

BEEFY STUFFED POBLANOS

4 SERVINGS (2 HALVES) // 45 MINUTES

This recipe works perfectly with ground beef or with vegetarian frozen crumbles.

4 large poblano peppers

1 16-ounce can refried beans

1 pound extra-lean ground beef or 12 ounces vegetarian frozen crumbles

¾ cup salsa

1 cup (4 oz.) mozzarella cheese, shredded

1 Preheat oven to 350 degrees F. Line a 9 × 13-inch baking dish with foil. Cut around the stems of the peppers and remove. Cut peppers in half and remove the seeds and inner membranes. Place halves cut side up in baking dish. Spread 3 tablespoons of refried beans in each pepper half.

2 In a large pan, brown meat until fully cooked, breaking up chunks with a wooden spoon. (If using vegetarian crumbles, just cook until warm.) Stir in salsa and turn off heat.

3 Divide meat mixture among pepper halves. Bake for 30 minutes. Remove from oven.

4 Top each pepper half with 2 tablespoons shredded cheese. Return to oven for 2–3 minutes to melt cheese.

Per serving (with ground beef): 352 calories, 12 g fat, 24 g total carbohydrate, 6 g dietary fiber, 37 g protein

+ CARBS Serve with 1 cup **Cilantro-Lime Brown Rice** (p. 121) for 72 g total carbohydrate.

If you have leftover filling, wrap it in a whole-wheat tortilla with some cooked rice to make a tasty burrito.

DQS COUNT (per serving)   VEGETABLES 1   LEAN MEATS & FISH 1   DAIRY 1

BLACK BEAN & CHEDDAR BURGERS

4 SERVINGS // 30 MINUTES

When you have the time, the best vegetarian burgers are made fresh. High in protein and fiber, these cheeseburgers are tasty enough for everyone to enjoy. The cheese is mixed into the patty for added flavor in every bite.

2 15-ounce cans black beans, drained and rinsed

1 egg

½ cup plain oatmeal (quick or old-fashioned)

2 teaspoons ground cumin

½ teaspoon cayenne pepper

½ cup (2 oz.) cheddar cheese, shredded

2 tablespoons cilantro, chopped (optional)

½ teaspoon extra-virgin olive oil (or olive-oil cooking spray)

whole-wheat buns (optional)

1 In a small food processor or blender, combine 1 can of beans, egg, oatmeal, cumin, and cayenne. Pulse to process until nearly smooth, stirring between pulses as needed with spatula or wooden spoon. Transfer mixture to a large bowl and add remaining beans, cheese, and cilantro, if desired. Stir well to mix.

2 Divide the mixture in the bowl into two equal portions. (This helps to make 4 equal-sized burgers with less guesswork.) Spread oil in the bottom of a large nonstick skillet, or mist lightly with cooking spray.

3 Use a plastic spatula to scoop up half of one portion of burger mixture and place it in the pan. Use the spatula to form it into a patty about 4 inches across. Form one more burger, and then repeat this step with the remaining half of the black-bean mixture.

4 Cook over medium heat for 8–10 minutes, turning halfway through, until crisp on both sides. Serve with lettuce, greens, pickles, or other desired toppings.

Per serving: 280 calories, 7 g fat, 37 g total carbohydrate, 13 g dietary fiber, 17 g protein

+ CARBS Serve on a whole-wheat bun for 68 g total carbohydrate.

DQS COUNT (per serving)   VEGETABLES   1 (1 legumes)

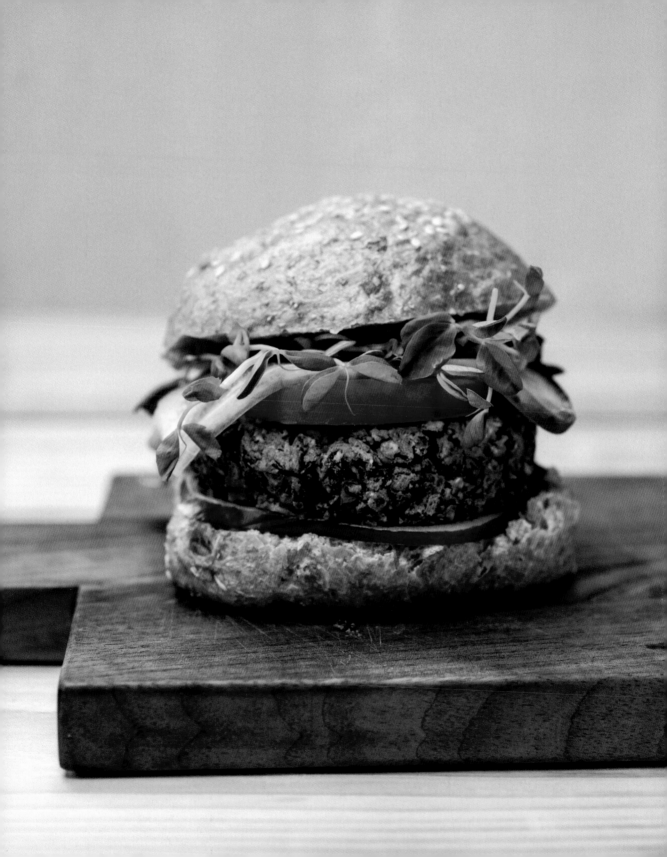

QUINOA & CHICKPEA SALAD

4 SERVINGS // 25 MINUTES

This dish was inspired by the flavors of tabbouleh, a classic Mediterranean salad. Quinoa and chickpeas (garbanzo beans) are used in place of cracked wheat, boosting fiber and protein content. Lots of fresh parsley is key to the salad's fresh flavor; cherry tomatoes and red onion add color and texture. Leftovers are even better the next day.

1 cup quinoa, rinsed and drained

2 cups water

2 tablespoons extra-virgin olive oil

3 tablespoons lemon juice

½ teaspoon salt

1 15-ounce can chickpeas (garbanzo beans), rinsed and drained

⅓ cup red onion, chopped

1 pint (10 oz.) grape tomatoes, quartered

1 cup flat-leaf parsley leaves, chopped

1 Combine quinoa and water in a small pot and simmer for 15 minutes or until water is absorbed. Set aside to cool.

2 In a large mixing bowl stir together olive oil, lemon juice, and salt. Add chickpeas, onion, tomatoes, and parsley to bowl and mix. Stir in cooled quinoa.

Per serving: 350 calories, 11 g fat, 55 g total carbohydrate, 11 g dietary fiber, 13 g protein

 TIP

Save 15 minutes by using 3 cups precooked quinoa.

DQS COUNT (per serving)   VEGETABLES 1 (1 legumes)   WHOLE GRAINS 1

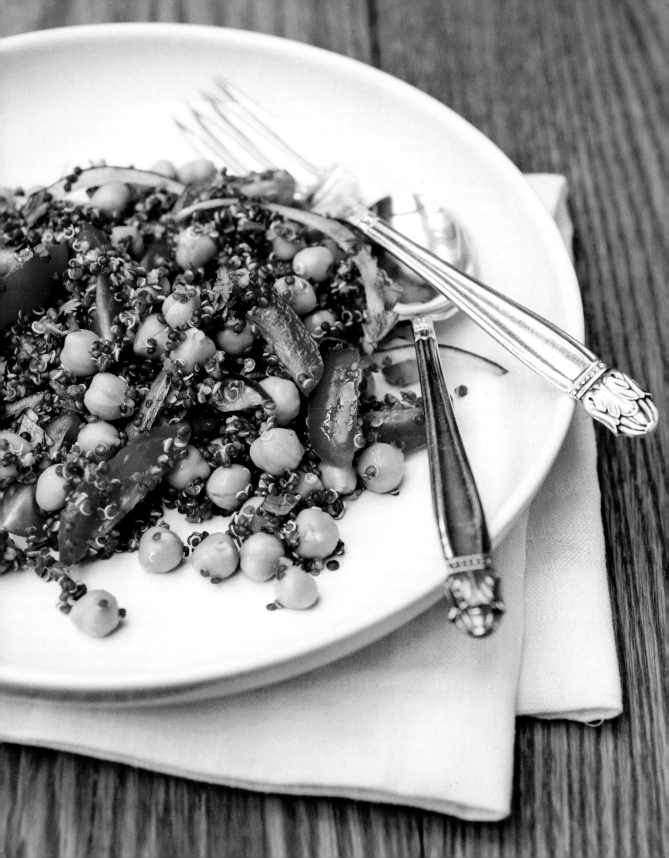

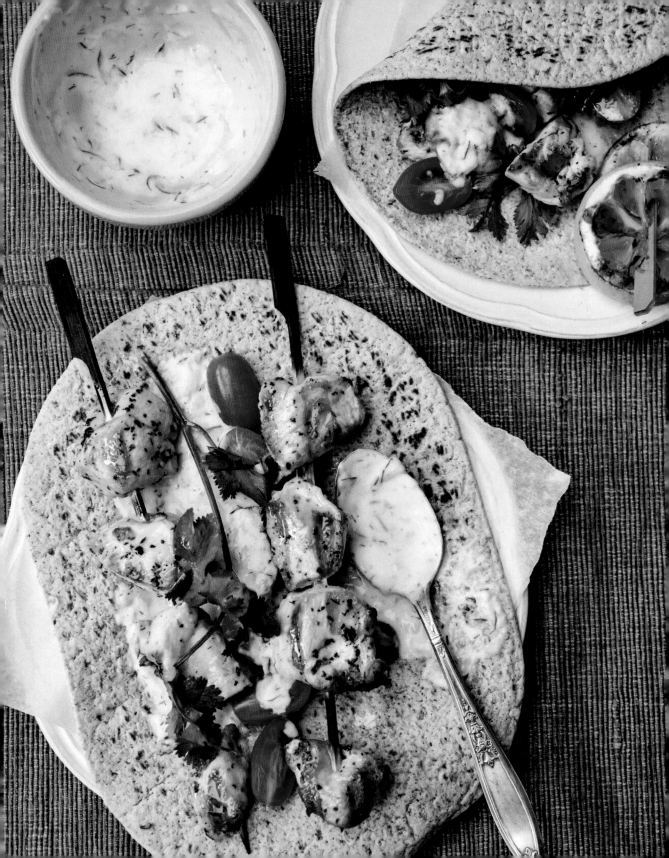

CHICKEN SOUVLAKI

4 SERVINGS // 30 MINUTES

An olive oil, herb, and lemon marinade makes chicken shine in this classic Greek dish. Serve with tzatziki sauce for a genuine souvlaki experience.

2 tablespoons extra-virgin olive oil

1 tablespoon lemon juice

2 teaspoons red wine vinegar

1½ teaspoons dried thyme

1½ teaspoons dried oregano

¼ teaspoon salt

¼ teaspoon black pepper

1 pound boneless, skinless chicken breasts

4 6.5-inch whole-wheat pitas

In a large mixing bowl, stir together olive oil, lemon juice, vinegar, thyme, oregano, salt, and pepper.

Cut chicken into 1½-inch cubes, place in marinade, and stir to coat. Marinate for 10–20 minutes.

Preheat indoor or outdoor grill to medium-high heat. Thread chicken on skewers and cook for 4 minutes on each side, or until just cooked through. Serve on whole-wheat pita and garnish with tomatoes and fresh herbs, if desired.

Per serving (with whole-wheat pita): 351 calories, 10 g fat, 36 g total carbohydrate, 5 g dietary fiber, 32 g protein

DQS COUNT (per serving) WHOLE GRAINS 1   LEAN MEATS & FISH 1

TZATZIKI SAUCE

10 SERVINGS (¼ CUP) // 40 MINUTES PLUS 1 HOUR TO CHILL

2 cups (2 to 3 medium) cucumber, peeled, seeded, and grated

¼ teaspoon salt

2 cups plain 2% Greek yogurt

4 cloves garlic, minced

2 tablespoons fresh dill, finely chopped

1½ tablespoons lemon juice

salt

Spread the grated cucumber on several layers of paper towels and sprinkle with salt. Let stand for 30 minutes.

In a medium bowl, combine cucumber, yogurt, garlic, dill, and lemon juice; stir to blend. Add salt to taste and refrigerate at least 1 hour before serving.

Per serving: 38 calories, 1 g fat, 3 g total carbohydrate, 0 g dietary fiber, 5 g protein

DQS COUNT (per serving) DAIRY 1

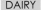

LENTIL SALAD

2 SERVINGS (1½ CUPS) // 30 MINUTES PLUS 1 HOUR TO CHILL

1 cup green
  or brown lentils

1 tablespoon
  Dijon mustard

1 tablespoon
  extra-virgin olive oil

2 tablespoons
  white vinegar

¼ teaspoon salt

⅓ cup red onion, minced

½ cup carrots, minced

1 Rinse lentils in a wire strainer, sorting through to remove gravel and other debris. Place lentils in a pot and cover with cold water. Bring to a simmer and cook for 20–25 minutes, or until lentils are al dente, not mushy. Rinse in a strainer under cold running water and drain well.

2 Whisk together mustard, olive oil, vinegar, and salt in a large bowl. Add minced onion and carrots and cooked lentils. Stir gently to mix.

3 Chill salad for at least 1 hour, and stir gently before serving.

Makes about 3 cups.

Per serving: 326 calories, 7 g fat, 47 g total carbohydrate, 24 g dietary fiber, 21 g protein

DQS COUNT (per serving)   VEGETABLES   1 (1 legumes)

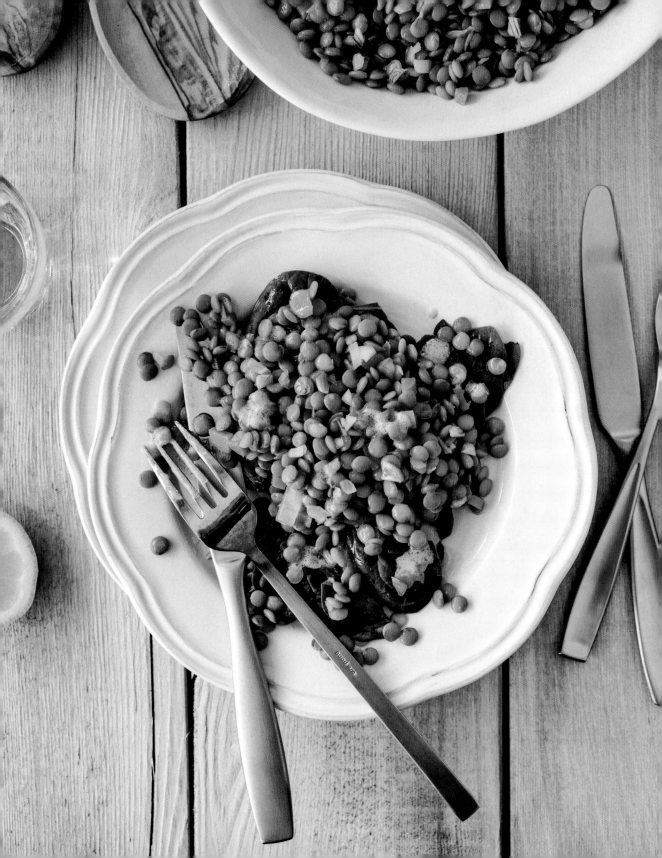

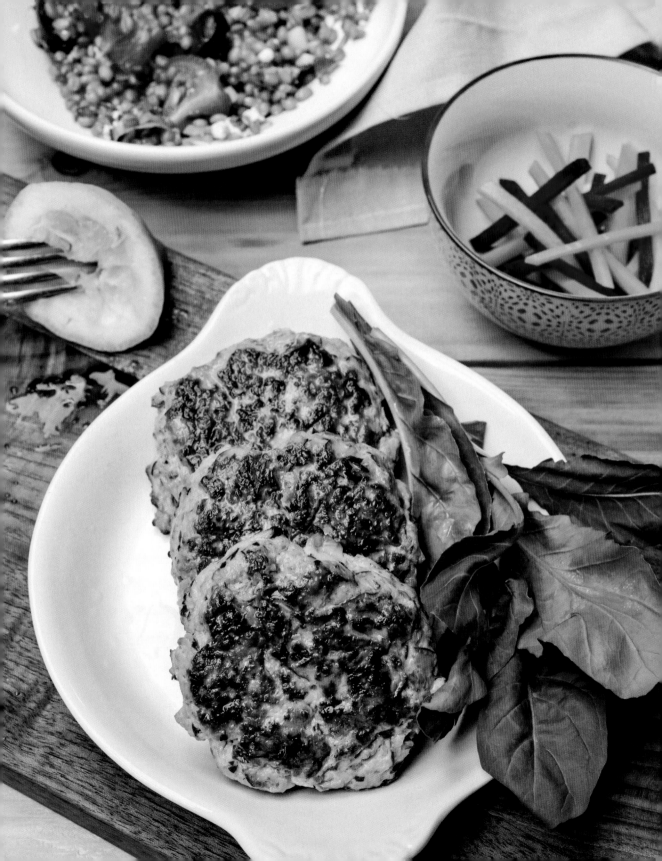

LEAN TURKEY BURGERS

4 SERVINGS // 20 MINUTES

Lean meats often make for a dry, tasteless burger, but fattier meat doesn't give you the high quality you want for your diet. The solution: Add moisture with grated vegetables. The result is a flavorful burger without the extra fat and calories.

4 white button mushrooms

1 medium zucchini

⅓ cup sweet onion, minced

2 tablespoons flat-leaf parsley, chopped

½ teaspoon salt

⅛ teaspoon black pepper

1¼ pounds 99% lean ground turkey breast

cooking spray

1 Using a box grater, finely grate mushrooms and zucchini into a large bowl. Mince onion and parsley, and add to bowl. Add salt and pepper, and gently mix in turkey until mixture is uniform. Form into 4 patties.

2 Lightly coat a large nonstick pan with cooking spray and heat over medium flame. When hot, add turkey patties and cook for 5–6 minutes on each side or until internal temperature reaches 160 degrees F.

Per serving: 177 calories, 1 g fat, 3 g total carbohydrate, 1 g dietary fiber, 35 g protein

 CARBS Serve on a whole-wheat bun for 34 g total carbohydrate.

DQS COUNT (per serving)   LEAN MEATS & FISH   1

STEAK WITH CHARRED CORN SALSA

4 SERVINGS // 45 MINUTES PLUS 3 HOURS TO MARINATE

The charred corn gives an incredible sweetness to the salsa. Substitute chicken for the steak if you prefer and use your favorite seasoning.

1 pound lean flank steak or top round

½ cup Worcestershire sauce

steak seasoning

CORN SALSA

1 large ear of corn (1 cup kernels)

1 cup red onion, finely chopped

1 jalapeño pepper, seeded and finely chopped

⅛ teaspoon salt

1 cup cherry or grape tomatoes, quartered

1 tablespoon white vinegar

1 tablespoon lime juice

1 To prepare lean steak, place in a glass or ceramic container, coat with Worcestershire sauce, cover with plastic wrap, and refrigerate for at least 3 hours.

2 Place corn on end in a large bowl and carefully use a paring knife to cut kernels from cob. Spread kernels in a single layer on a dry nonstick skillet. Cook over medium-high heat for 15–20 minutes, stirring every 5 minutes, until kernels are charred.

3 Transfer charred corn to a large mixing bowl and add onion, jalapeño, salt, tomatoes, vinegar, and lime juice. Stir to blend. Refrigerate salsa while preparing meat.

4 Season both sides of steak with steak seasoning before grilling to desired doneness.

5 Serve steak with charred corn salsa heaped on top.

Per serving (with London broil beef): 244 calories, 9 g fat, 12 g total carbohydrate, 2 g dietary fiber, 27 g protein

DQS COUNT (per serving)   VEGETABLES 1   LEAN MEATS & FISH 1

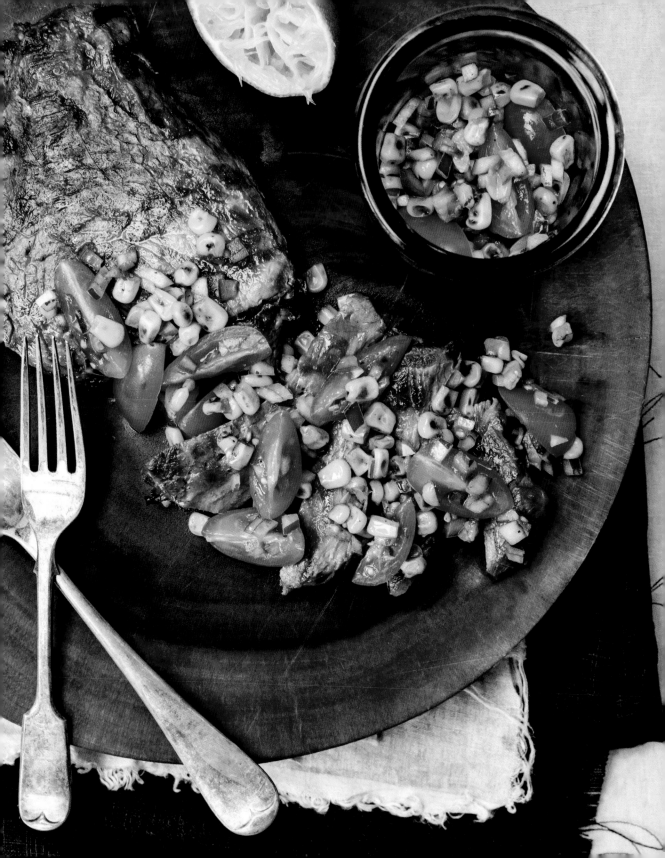

RASPBERRY & FETA SALAD WITH WHEAT BERRIES

2 SERVINGS // 10 MINUTES

Cooked grains atop a salad provide a boost of minerals and complex carbohydrates; they also add a delightful chewy texture and soak up flavors from whatever dressing you enjoy. This salad pairs sweet raspberries with salty feta cheese and red onion.

6 cups (5 oz.) mixed salad greens, loosely packed

1 cup *cooked* wheat berries or barley

1 cup raspberries

½ cup (4 oz.) feta cheese, crumbled

½ cup red onion, thinly sliced

1 | Divide salad greens between two plates, and top evenly with cooked grains, raspberries, feta, and onion.

Per serving: 261 calories, 7 g fat, 44 g total carbohydrate, 7 g dietary fiber, 11 g protein

 TIP

Swap out the onion for another crunchy ingredient such as carrots, jicama, or celery.

DQS COUNT (per serving)   FRUITS ½   VEGETABLES 1   WHOLE GRAINS 1   DAIRY 1

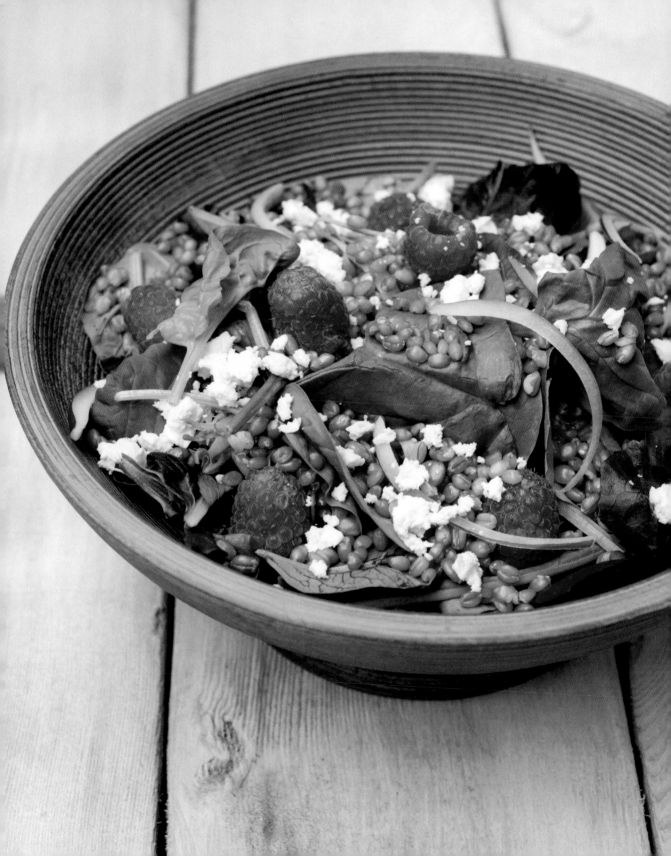

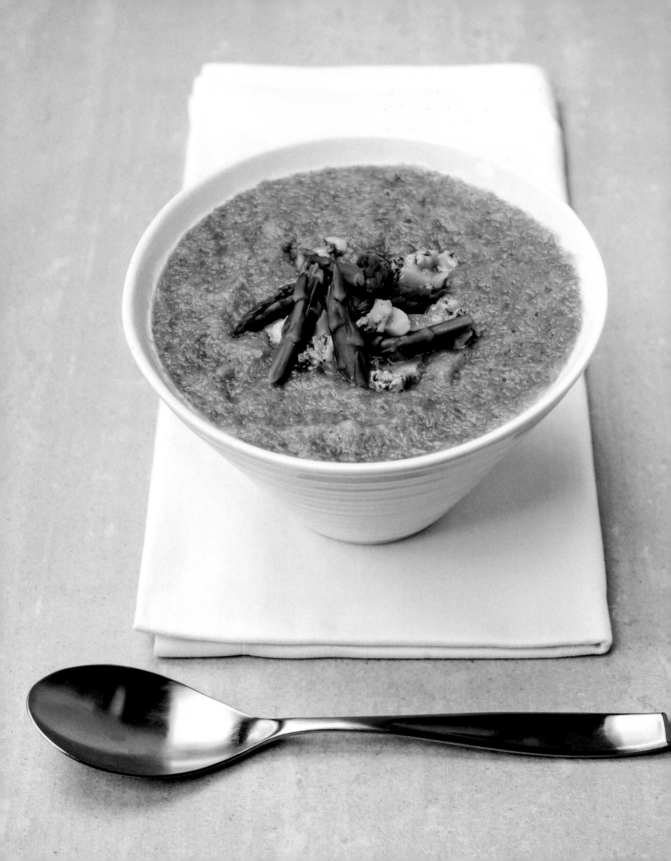

ASPARAGUS & BLUE CHEESE SOUP

2 SERVINGS // 25 MINUTES

This creamy soup gets a punch of flavor from the blue cheese. But don't be fooled by the taste; it's quite low in calories and fat. Enjoy this as a delicious starter, or pair it with beef or steak.

1½ cups vegetable broth

1½ cups cauliflower, finely chopped

8 ounces (½ bunch) asparagus, chopped with tips reserved

1 clove garlic, chopped

2 tablespoons (1 oz.) blue cheese, crumbled

1 Place broth, cauliflower, asparagus (except the tips), and garlic in a small saucepan and bring to a boil for 8 minutes.

2 Transfer mixture to blender and puree until smooth. Return to saucepan and add asparagus tips. Boil for 8 minutes more, then stir in the cheese, reserving a bit to garnish each bowl of soup.

Per serving: 68 calories, 2 g fat, 9 g total carbohydrate, 4 g dietary fiber, 5 g protein

DQS COUNT (per serving) VEGETABLES 2 DAIRY ½

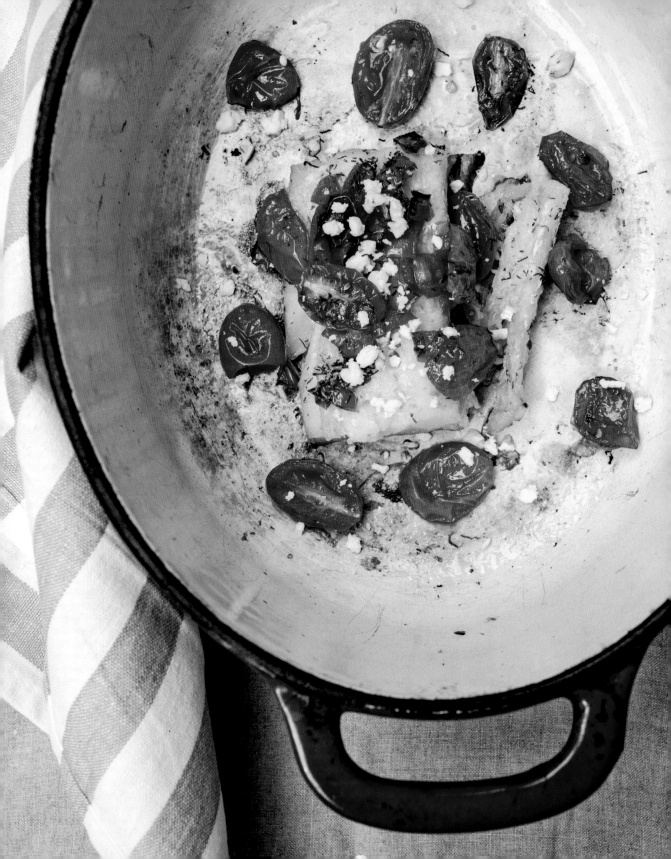

COD WITH TOMATOES, DILL & FETA

3 SERVINGS // 20 MINUTES

cooking spray

1 pound cod

salt and pepper

¾ cup canned petite diced tomatoes, drained

1 plum tomato, chopped

¼ teaspoon dried dill

½ cup (4 oz.) feta cheese, crumbled

1 Preheat oven to 425 degrees F. Lightly mist an 8 × 8-inch or 9 × 9-inch baking pan with cooking spray and place cod on it. Season with salt and pepper to taste.

2 Spoon diced tomatoes on top of fish, and top with chopped fresh tomato. Sprinkle dill on top of tomatoes.

3 Bake for 15 minutes, or until fish flakes easily with a fork. Divide into 4 portions and top with feta before serving.

Per serving: 188 calories, 5 g fat, 4 g total carbohydrate, 1 g dietary fiber, 31 g protein

+ CARBS Serve with **Garlic & Butter Brown Rice** for 52 g total carbohydrate.

DQS COUNT (per serving)   VEGETABLES ½   LEAN MEATS & FISH 1   DAIRY ½

WHEAT BERRY SALAD WITH FETA & OLIVES

4 SERVINGS // 1 HOUR, 10 MINUTES

3 cups water

pinch of salt

1 cup wheat berries, rinsed and drained

½ cup red onion, chopped

2 large tomatoes, chopped

½ cup parsley (curly or flat-leaf), chopped

¼ cup kalamata olives, chopped

½ cup (4 oz.) feta cheese, crumbled

2 teaspoons red wine vinegar

¼ teaspoon black pepper

1 Combine water with a pinch of salt in a medium saucepan and bring to a boil over medium-high heat. Add wheat berries, reduce heat, cover, and simmer for 60 minutes or until tender but chewy. Remove from heat, strain water, and transfer wheat berries into a bowl. Refrigerate wheat berries while other ingredients are prepared.

2 In a large mixing bowl, combine all remaining ingredients and mix gently to combine. Once cool, fold in the wheat berries and chill until serving.

Per serving: 233 calories, 7 g fat, 28 g total carbohydrate, 5 g dietary fiber, 8 g protein

If you have 3 cups of cooked wheat berries in the fridge, you can put this salad together in 10 minutes.

DQS COUNT (per serving)   VEGETABLES ½   WHOLE GRAINS 1   DAIRY 1

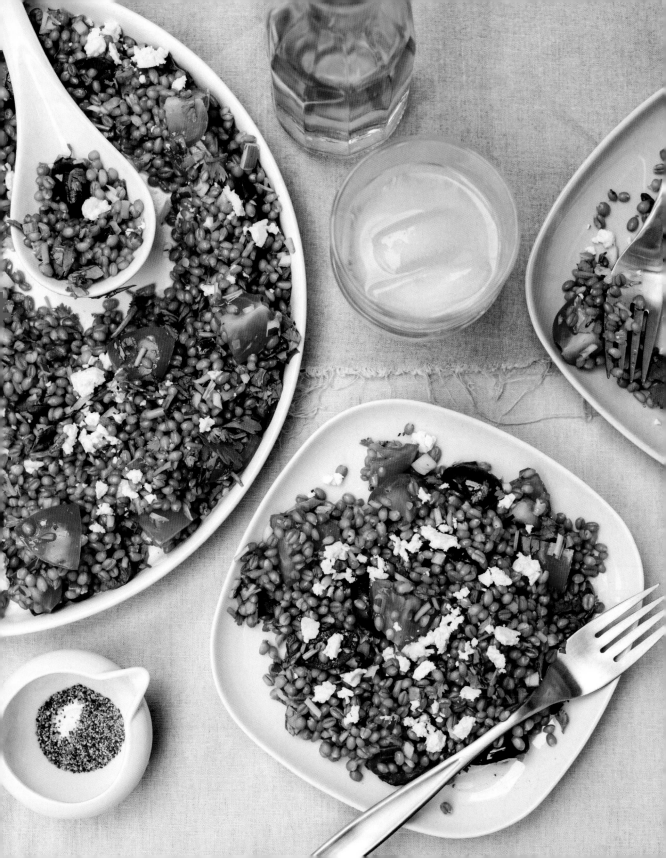

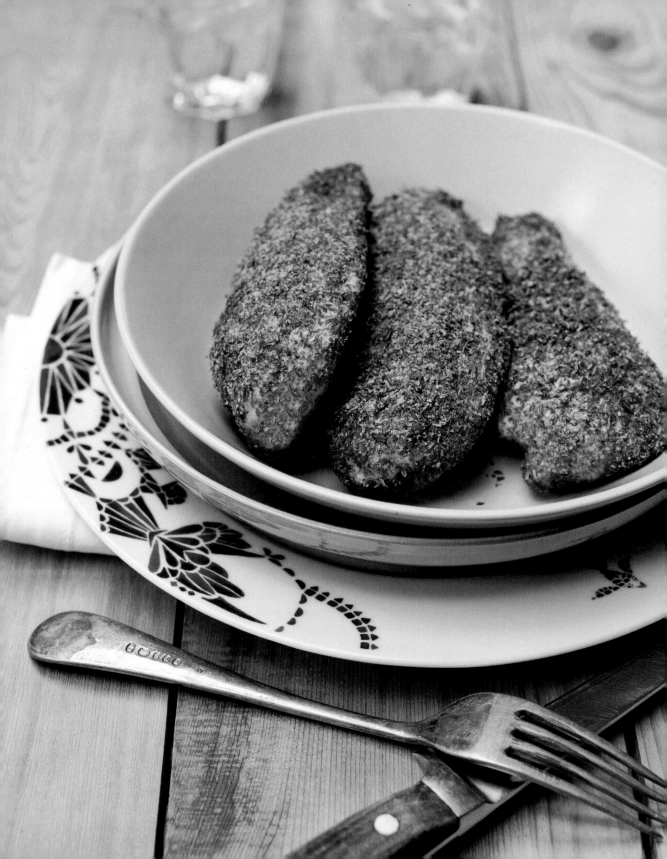

FLAXSEED & HERB–CRUSTED CHICKEN

3 SERVINGS // 30 MINUTES

The crisp flaxseed crust keeps the chicken wonderfully moist inside. You can use golden or brown flaxseed; the only difference is color.

cooking spray

¼ cup ground golden flaxseed

2 tablespoons dried onion flakes

½ teaspoon each dried dill, dried oregano, garlic powder, and salt

⅛ teaspoon black pepper

2 tablespoons egg substitute or 1 egg, beaten

1 pound boneless, skinless chicken breasts

1 Preheat oven to 400 degrees F. Line a baking sheet with foil and place wire rack on top of it. Mist rack lightly with cooking spray.

2 In a shallow, wide bowl combine flaxseed, onion flakes, dill, oregano, garlic, salt, and pepper. Place egg substitute or beaten egg in a separate bowl.

3 Dip one chicken breast into egg, allow excess to drip off, and press each side into flaxseed mixture to coat. Place on wire rack on prepared baking sheet. Repeat with each chicken breast.

4 Bake for 20 minutes or until a thermometer inserted in thickest part of chicken reads 160 degrees F.

Per serving: 203 calories, 5 g fat, 6 g total carbohydrate, 4 g dietary fiber, 37 g protein

If you don't have a wire rack, you can cook the chicken on a baking sheet alone.

DQS COUNT (per serving)   LEAN MEATS & FISH 1   NUTS & SEEDS 1

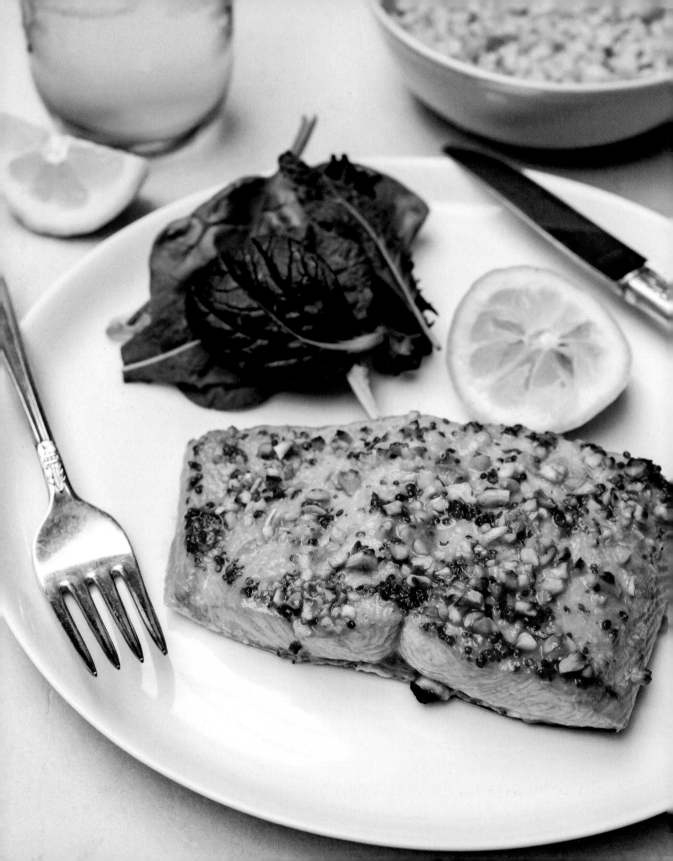

CASHEW-CRUSTED SALMON

3 SERVINGS // 15 MINUTES

A few simple ingredients are all you need for an amazing seafood entrée at home. This recipe balances tangy mustard with a touch of sweetness and a crunchy cashew crust.

- 1 **pound wild salmon fillets**
- 1 **teaspoon honey**
- 1 **teaspoon whole-grain mustard**
  pinch of salt
- 3 **tablespoons (1 oz.) cashews**

1 Preheat broiler to high heat. Line a baking sheet with foil, and lay salmon on it skin side down.

2 In a small bowl, stir together honey, mustard, and salt. Spread mixture evenly on fish.

3 Use the back of a wooden spoon or the side of a chef's knife to crush cashews. Sprinkle over salmon.

4 Broil until salmon flakes easily with a fork in the thickest part, which can take 5–10 minutes depending on your broiler and the thickness of the fillet.

Per serving: 339 calories, 16 g fat, 5 g total carbohydrate, 0 g dietary fiber, 43 g protein

WILD VERSUS FARMED SALMON

Wild salmon has a far better flavor and contains fewer environmental contaminants than farmed salmon. Compared with wild salmon, farmed salmon has been shown to be contaminated with up to ten times as many environmental toxins, such as polychlorinated biphenyls (PCBs) and dioxin. Many of these toxins have been labeled probable carcinogens by health authorities. Farmed salmon are fattier than their wild counterparts, and the toxins accumulate in the fat. Also, the pellets of food used to feed farmed salmon have been shown to be highly contaminated with environmental toxins.

If you see fish that is labeled "Atlantic salmon," it comes from a farm. We recommend that you don't eat any Atlantic, or farmed, salmon and choose only fish that is clearly labeled "wild." The best pick for sustainability, low levels of contamination, and health is Alaskan wild salmon, followed by wild salmon caught in British Columbia or the Yukon.

DQS COUNT (per serving)   LEAN MEATS & FISH 1   NUTS & SEEDS ½

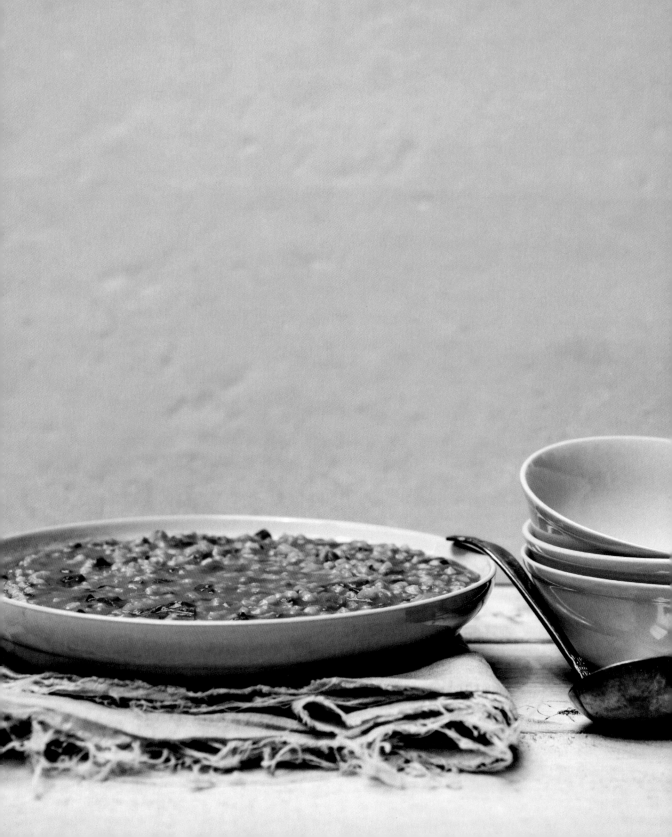

TOMATO-BASIL SOUP WITH PEARL BARLEY

4 SERVINGS (1½ CUPS) // 35 MINUTES

½ tablespoon extra-virgin olive oil

3 cloves garlic, minced

5 cups water

1 cup pearl barley, rinsed and drained

1 6-ounce can organic tomato paste

2 cups Swiss chard (or spinach), finely chopped

1 teaspoon salt

1 handful fresh basil, shredded

1 In a large pot, heat olive oil and garlic over medium heat and cook until fragrant.

2 Add water and barley, and raise heat to high. When water boils, turn down to low and cover. Simmer for 15 minutes.

3 Add tomato paste, chard, and salt, and stir to dissolve tomato paste. Simmer for 15 minutes longer. Add basil for the last 2 minutes, then remove from heat and serve.

Makes about 6 cups.

Per serving: 204 calories, 2 fat, 45 g total carbohydrate, 9 g dietary fiber, 6 g protein

DQS COUNT (per serving) VEGETABLES 1 WHOLE GRAINS 1

TURKEY MEATBALLS & FETTUCCINE

8 SERVINGS // 1 HOUR

2 pounds 99% lean ground turkey breast

⅓ cup whole-wheat bread crumbs

2 eggs

3 cloves garlic, minced

1 tablespoon dried onion flakes

2 tablespoons fresh basil, chopped

½ teaspoon salt

¼ teaspoon black pepper

cooking spray

4 cups tomato-basil pasta sauce from a jar

1 pinch of salt

1 pound whole-wheat fettuccine

1 Combine ground turkey, bread crumbs, eggs, garlic, onion flakes, basil, salt, and pepper in a large bowl and mix well.

2 Coat a large nonstick skillet with cooking spray. Roll meat mixture into 40 2-inch balls and place a single layer in the skillet. (They usually have to be cooked in two batches.)

3 Brown over medium heat, using tongs or a wooden spoon to turn the meatballs so the outsides cook evenly.

4 Transfer meatballs to a large saucepan and pour in the tomato-basil sauce. Cover and simmer over a low flame for 40 minutes.

5 While the meatballs are cooking, fill a large saucepan with water and a pinch of salt. Bring to a boil over medium-high heat, then add fettucine. Cook 12–14 minutes or as directed on the package. Pour into a colander to drain.

6 Add about ¾ cup cooked fettucine to each plate and top with meatballs and sauce.

Per serving: 400 calories, 5 g fat, 55 g total carbohydrate, 8 g dietary fiber, 38 g protein

You can purchase a commercial brand of whole-wheat bread crumbs, such as 4C, or make your own with bread you have on hand.

DQS COUNT (per serving)   VEGETABLES 1   WHOLE GRAINS 1   LEAN MEATS & FISH 1

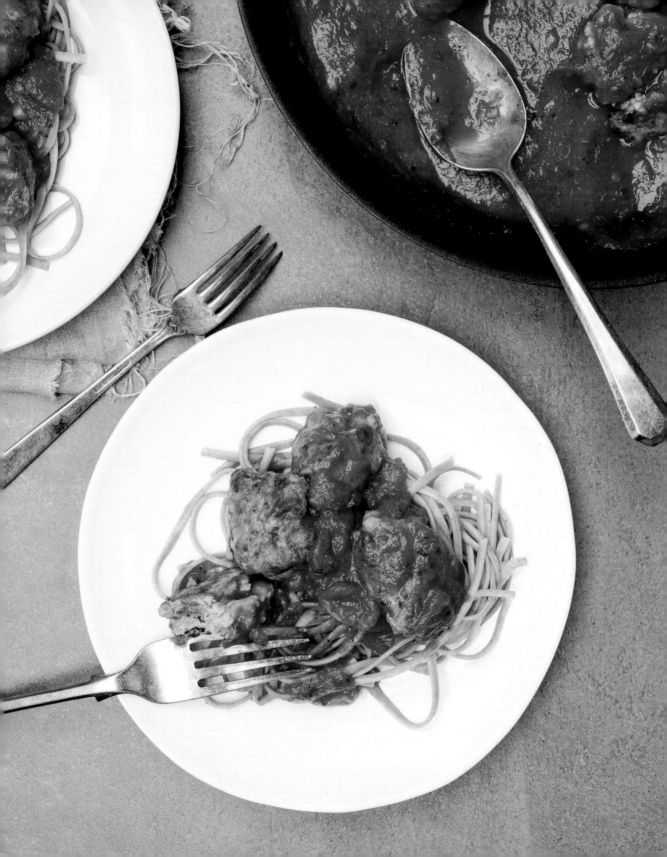

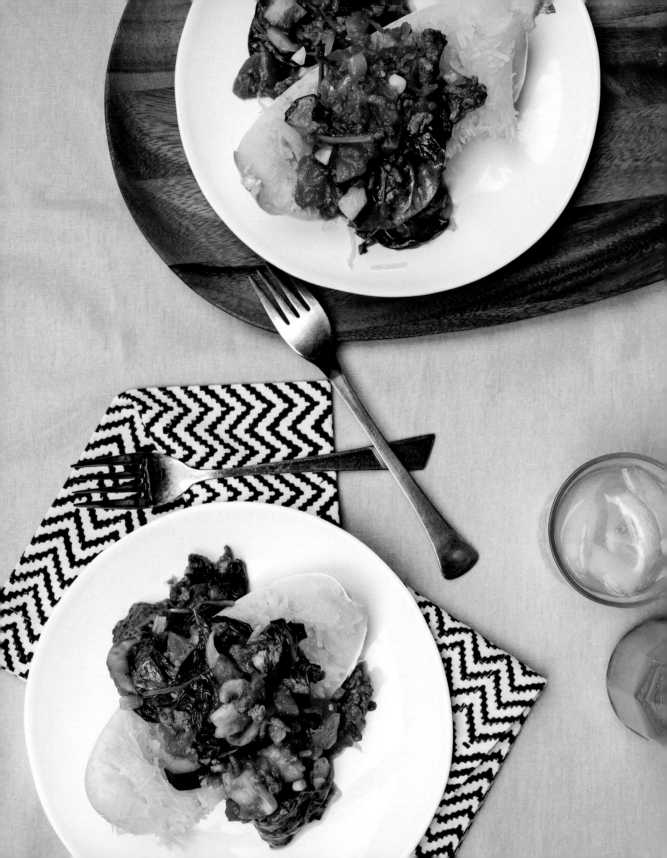

BEEF-VEGETABLE RAGU OVER SPAGHETTI SQUASH

2 SERVINGS // 40 MINUTES

You can serve any pasta dish atop spaghetti squash for a lower-carbohydrate, lower-calorie option. When you scoop out the cooked strands, it's easy to see how this squash got its name.

- 1 medium spaghetti squash
- ⅔ pound lean ground beef
- 4 cloves garlic
- 1 cup mushrooms, sliced
- 1 medium zucchini, cubed
- ½ yellow onion, chopped
- 1 14½-ounce can diced tomatoes (with liquid)
- ½ teaspoon dried basil
- ½ teaspoon red pepper flakes
- ¼ teaspoon salt
- 4 cups fresh baby spinach

1 Cut squash in half lengthwise and scrape out seeds. Wrap one half in a wet paper towel and microwave for 6 minutes or until flesh is tender and scrapes out easily with a fork. Repeat with other half. Keep warm.

2 While spaghetti squash is cooking, brown beef in a large nonstick skillet, breaking up the meat with a wooden spoon. When it is fully cooked, add garlic, mushrooms, zucchini, onion, tomatoes, basil, red pepper flakes, and salt.

3 Cover and simmer for 10 minutes. Stir in spinach and cook for 2 minutes longer, or until it wilts but retains a bright green color.

4 Split cooked spaghetti squash between two plates, which should be about 2 cups per serving. Top generously with ragu.

Per serving: 406 calories, 12 g fat, 38 g total carbohydrate, 7 g dietary fiber, 39 g protein

DQS COUNT (per serving)   VEGETABLES 3   LEAN MEATS & FISH 1

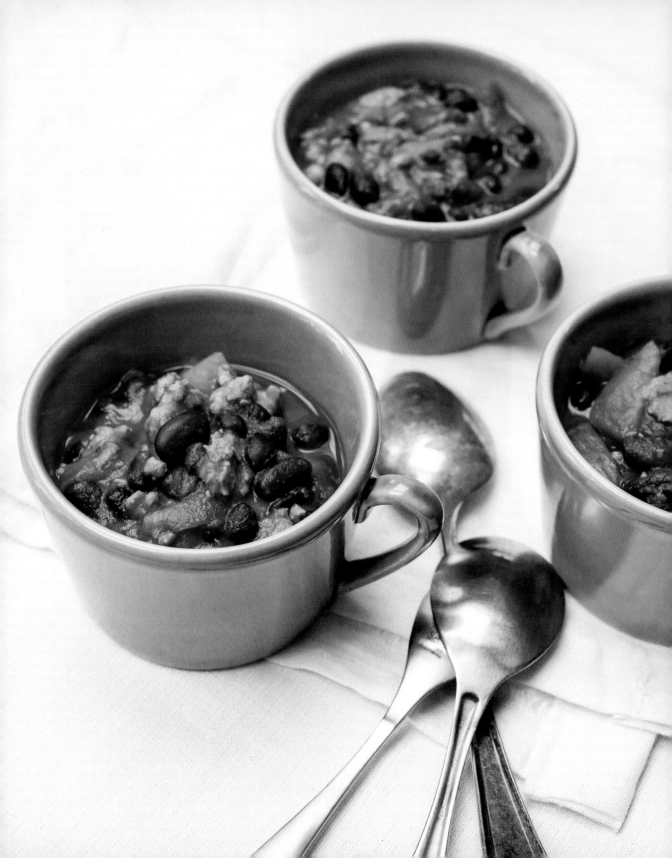

TWO-BEAN PUMPKIN CHILI

4 SERVINGS // 45 MINUTES

Canned pumpkin and a touch of cinnamon give this chili a unique fall flavor, but it is still traditional enough to be recognized as chili.

1 pound 93% lean ground turkey or beef (optional)

1 green pepper or poblano pepper, chopped

1 yellow onion, chopped

1½ cups water

1 cup canned pumpkin

1 15-ounce can dark red kidney beans, rinsed and drained

1 15-ounce can black beans, rinsed and drained

2 tablespoons tomato paste

2 teaspoons chili powder

½ teaspoon ground cayenne pepper

½ teaspoon ground cinnamon

½ teaspoon salt or to taste

1 If using meat, heat a saucepan over medium heat and add turkey or beef. Brown meat, breaking up with a wooden spoon or spatula. Drain any liquid.

2 Add all remaining ingredients to pot and stir to mix. Bring to a boil, then cover pot and turn heat to low. Simmer for 30 minutes, stirring occasionally to check thickness. Add more water if chili is too thick. If chili is too thin, remove cover and let liquid cook off a bit more.

Per serving (with 93% lean turkey): 408 calories, 10 g fat, 43 g carbohydrate, 14 g dietary fiber, 37 g protein

Per serving (without meat): 248 calories, 2 g fat, 43 g total carbohydrate, 14 g dietary fiber, 15 g protein

Make a double batch of chili and freeze half of it. Use quart-sized freezer bags to divide chili into smaller portions so it's easy to defrost one serving at a time.

DQS COUNT (per serving) VEGETABLES 2 (2 legumes) LEAN MEATS & FISH 1

SOLE WITH LEMON & CAPERS

2 SERVINGS // 15 MINUTES

12 ounces sole or flounder
salt and pepper
2 tablespoons
almond flour
1 teaspoon extra-virgin
olive oil or butter
½ lemon
1 tablespoon capers

Season fish with salt and pepper to taste, and sprinkle with almond flour.

Heat a skillet over medium heat and add oil or butter. When hot, add fish. Cook until fish is opaque around the edges and golden brown underneath. Then gently flip the fillets with a spatula. Cook on the second side for 2–3 minutes, until fish is opaque throughout. Transfer fish to plates and return skillet to heat.

Squeeze juice from lemon into the skillet and add capers, scraping with a spatula to loosen browned bits. Drizzle sauce over fish and serve.

Per serving: 214 calories, 8 g fat, 2 g total carbohydrate, 1 g dietary fiber, 33 g protein

DQS COUNT (per serving)   LEAN MEATS & FISH 1

GREEK POTATOES

6 SERVINGS // 30 MINUTES

5 pounds fingerling
or baby gold potatoes
2 tablespoons butter
2 tablespoons
Greek seasoning

Cut potatoes into 1-inch chunks and place in a microwave-safe dish with 2 inches of water.

Cover with a wet paper towel to trap steam. Microwave for 10 minutes or until tender.

Drain potatoes and transfer to a frying pan with butter and Greek seasoning (oregano may be used if Greek seasoning is not available). Cook over medium-high heat for 5 minutes, tossing occasionally, to brown in spots. Turn off heat and cover to keep warm.

Per serving: 314 calories, 4 g fat, 67 g total carbohydrate, 5 g dietary fiber, 8 g protein

DQS COUNT (per serving)   VEGETABLES 1

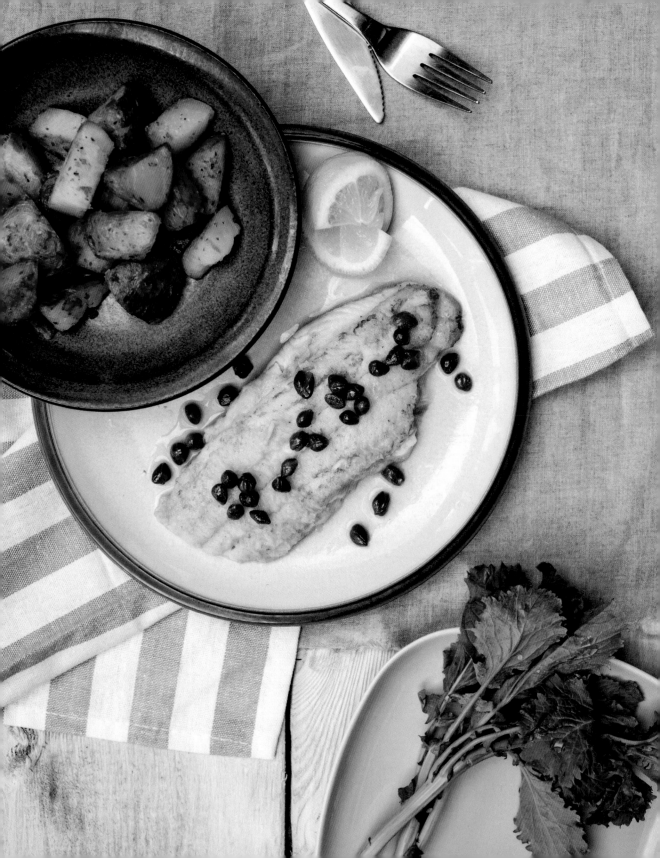

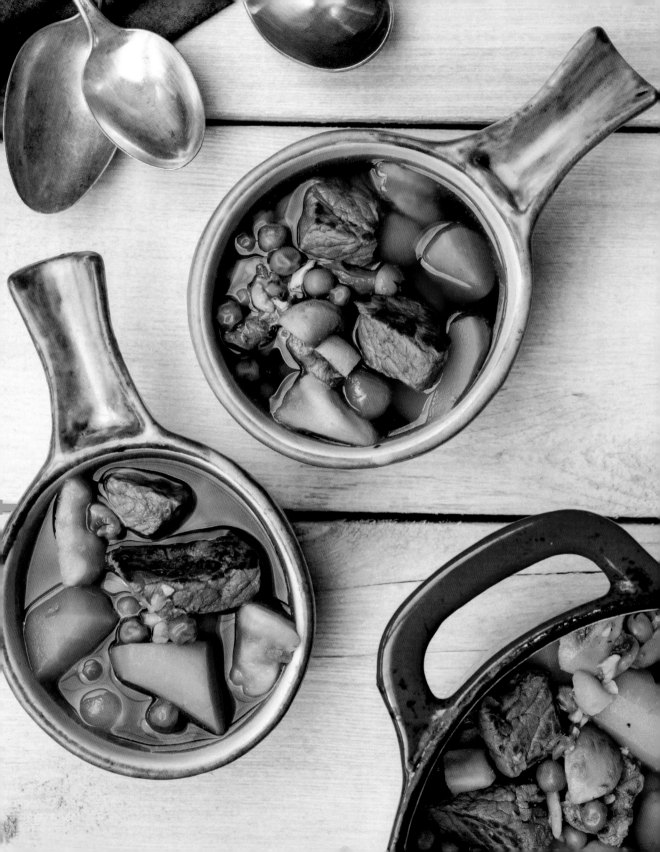

BEEF STEW WITH SWEET POTATOES

6 SERVINGS // 20 MINUTES PLUS 6 HOURS COOKING TIME

Substituting sweet potatoes for white potatoes boosts nutrition content, and this stew also has more veggies than many beef stew recipes. It has a great nutrient profile for a postworkout meal.

- 2 pounds lean beef, cubed
- 1½ cups beef broth
- 14 ounces *frozen* pearl onions, peeled
- 6 carrots, peeled and cut into 1-inch chunks
- 8 ounces cremini mushrooms, quartered
- 1 large (12 oz.) sweet potato, peeled and cubed
- 3 cloves garlic, minced
- 1 tablespoon Worcestershire sauce
- 2 teaspoons paprika
- ½ teaspoon seasoned salt
- ½ teaspoon ground black pepper
- ⅔ cup *frozen* peas

1 Combine all ingredients except peas in a slow cooker and stir. Cover and cook on low heat for 6 hours. Stir in peas when stew is done (the hot stew will cook them).

Per serving: 319 calories, 6 g fat, 29 g total carbohydrate, 6 g dietary fiber, 37 g protein

+ CARBS Double the sweet potato (to 1½ pounds) and use 1 cup of peas for 69 g total carbohydrate.

DQS COUNT (per serving)   VEGETABLES 2   LEAN MEATS & FISH 1

RED LENTILS WITH KALE & TOMATOES

4 SERVINGS (1½ CUPS) // 35 MINUTES

Nutritionally speaking, this is a powerhouse in a bowl! Reduce the portion size to serve as a smaller side with meat, chicken, or fish. Bump up the cayenne pepper if you want more kick.

2 teaspoons extra-virgin olive oil

6 cloves garlic, minced

1 cup onion, chopped

1 teaspoon cumin

½ teaspoon cayenne pepper

2 teaspoons paprika

2 14-ounce cans diced tomatoes (with liquid)

3 cups water

1½ cup red lentils

1 bunch kale, finely chopped

½ teaspoon salt

1 Place oil in a small pool in the center of a large skillet, and add garlic and onion. Cook over medium-low heat for 4 minutes or until soft.

2 Add cumin, cayenne, and paprika. Stir and cook for 1 minute to release flavors.

3 Add diced tomatoes with liquid, water, lentils, kale, and salt. Stir and raise heat to high. When mixture boils, reduce heat to low and cover. Simmer for 20 minutes or until liquid is absorbed.

Makes about 6 cups.

Per serving: 382 calories, 3 g fat, 66 g total carbohydrate, 17 g dietary fiber, 24 g protein

DQS COUNT (per serving)   VEGETABLES   2 (1 legumes)

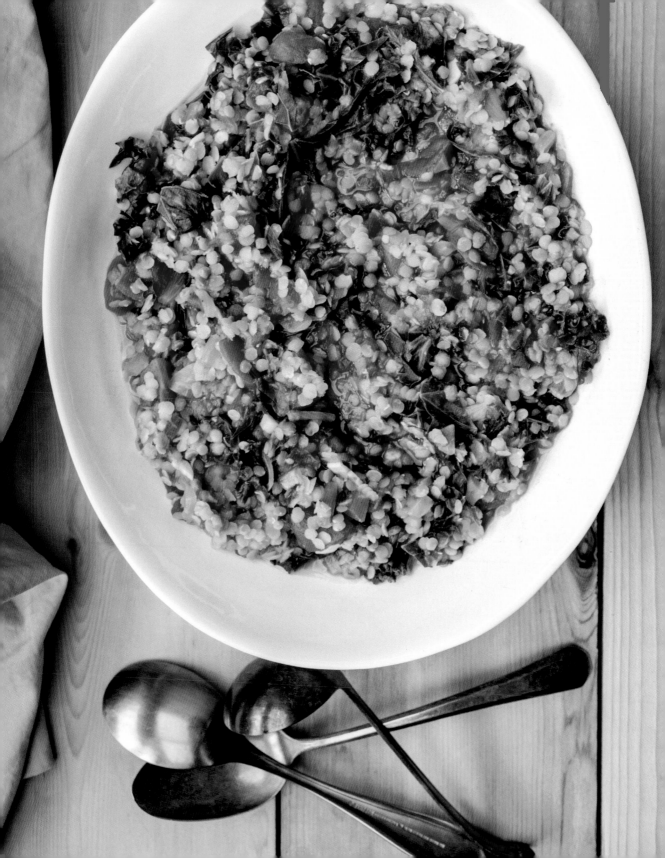

INDIVIDUAL MEAT LOAVES

8 SERVINGS // 1 HOUR, 15 MINUTES

Cute little meat loaves are both fun and practical—they cook faster than standard loaves and are perfectly portioned. Use a roasting pan or rack with holes, which allows the extra fat to drain.

2 pounds 93% lean ground beef

cooking spray

1 green bell pepper, finely chopped

½ cup onion, finely chopped

3 cloves garlic, minced

½ teaspoon dried oregano

½ teaspoon dried basil

¼ cup + 2 tablespoons whole-wheat bread crumbs

¾ teaspoon salt

½ teaspoon onion powder

½ teaspoon garlic powder

2 eggs

¼ cup organic ketchup

2 teaspoons Worcestershire sauce

1 Preheat oven to 375 degrees F.

2 Place beef in a large bowl and use a spatula to break it up so it will come to room temperature.

3 Spray a large skillet with cooking spray and add chopped peppers and onion. Cook over medium heat until vegetables start to soften, 4–5 minutes. Add garlic, oregano, and basil; cook for 1 minute longer and turn off heat. Let vegetables cool.

4 Sprinkle bread crumbs, salt, onion powder, and garlic powder over the meat and mix with your hands to combine. Add eggs and cooled vegetables and mix until well blended. (Do not overmix, or meat loaves will be tough.) Form mixture into 8 equal balls or ovals and place on a rack or roasting pan with holes.

5 Combine ketchup and Worcestershire sauce in a small bowl and brush the tops and sides of loaves with sauce. Bake for 60 minutes, or until a meat thermometer shows an internal temperature of 165 degrees F.

Per serving: 229 calories, 9 g fat, 9 g total carbohydrate, 1 g dietary fiber, 26 g protein

(See **Sour Cream & Onion Mashed Cauliflower** recipe on p. 168)

DQS COUNT (per serving)   LEAN MEATS & FISH   1

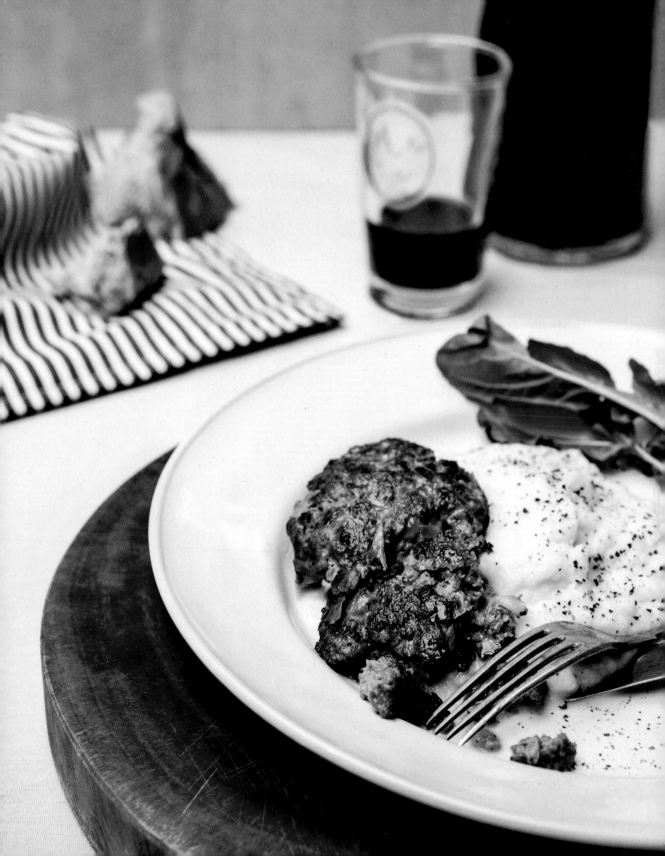

SOUR CREAM & ONION MASHED CAULIFLOWER

8 SERVINGS // 15 MINUTES (v) (See photo on p. 167)

Serve this dish with meat loaf or steak, and you could fool anyone into thinking it is whipped potatoes. It's incredibly delicious and satisfying and great for those times when you want fewer carbs. Don't count on having leftovers.

1	head cauliflower, chopped
½	teaspoon salt
1	teaspoon onion powder
¼	cup sour cream
	black pepper

1 Bring a pot of water to a boil and add cauliflower. Cover and boil until very tender, then drain all the liquid away in a colander.

2 Transfer cauliflower to a small food processor or blender, add remaining ingredients, and pulse until smooth. Use a rubber spatula periodically to press out any lumps.

Per serving: 89 calories, 5 g fat, 8 g total carbohydrate, 3 g dietary fiber, 3 g protein

DQS COUNT (per serving)   VEGETABLES 1   DAIRY ½

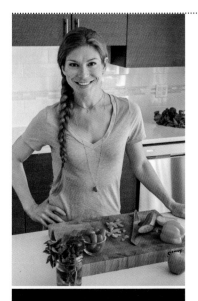

VARIETY WITHOUT HASSLE

Consistency is important when it comes to diet and meal timing. However, if you eat the same thing over and over, you will likely become bored with your diet, and your limited nutritional intake may compromise your performance. You'll gain the widest array of nutrients if you vary your meal choices instead of eating the same meals day after day. Furthermore, when you have varied healthful meal options, you're less likely to turn to junk food to break the monotony. Try making subtle changes to your favorite meals:

+ **Branch out in the produce department.** Instead of always eating just apples and bananas, grab some grapes, kiwi, oranges, or mangoes when they are in season.

+ **Vary your veggies.** Instead of having the same salad each day, mix things up by working in an array of greens such as spinach, radicchio, arugula, or shredded cabbage.

+ **Boost flavor with herbs.** Fresh herbs such as basil, oregano, cilantro, and dill make delicious additions. Add fresh cilantro to a green salad or scrambled eggs, top baked fish or cooked carrots with dill, or finish your tomato sauce with a handful of fresh oregano and basil.

+ **Use premixed spice blends.** You don't have to be a professional chef to season food well. Try Greek, Moroccan, Italian, Creole, or Cajun blends to flavor your proteins and make vegetables more interesting. Our favorite blends are from Savory Spice Shop (http://www.savoryspiceshop.com/spice-blends).

+ **Change things up with flavored olive oils and vinegars.** Drizzle them over cooked pasta or grains, mix them with vegetables before roasting, or use them to dress your salad greens with flair. For dozens of delicious options check out the Rocky Mountain Olive Oil Company (http://rockymountainoliveoil.com). Be sure to try the garlic olive oil.

THE ATHLETE WHO LOVES TO COOK

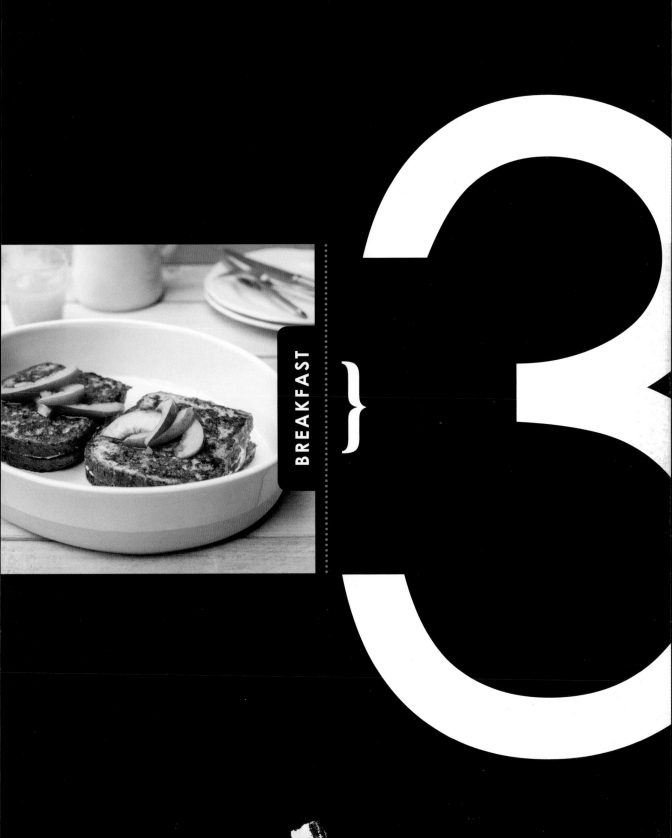

BREAKFAST

3

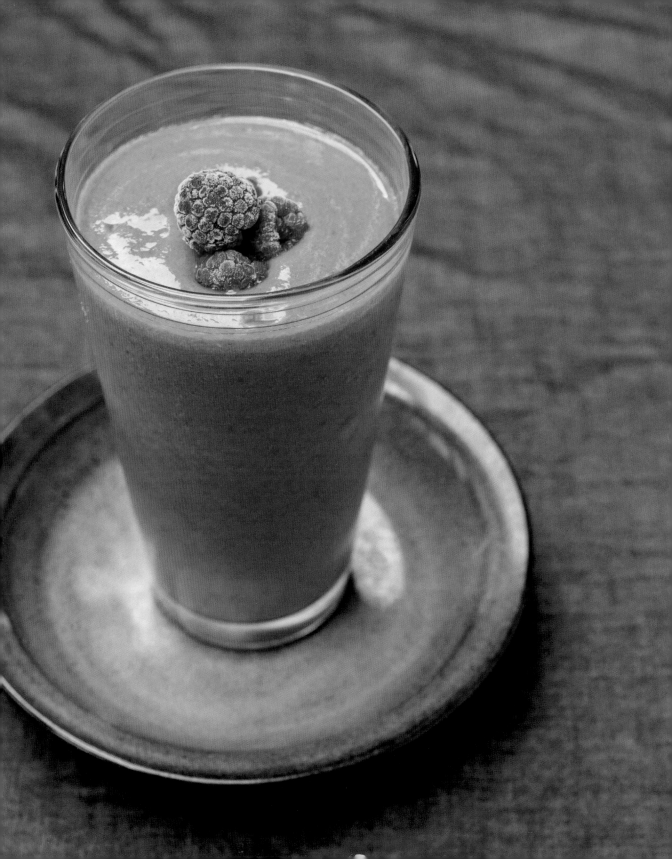

RASPBERRY-PEAR SMOOTHIE

1 SERVING // 5 MINUTES PLUS 1 HOUR FOR ROASTING BEETS

Beets are rich in nitrates, which increase your body's oxygen usage and aid your endurance performance. By adding beets to this raspberry smoothie, you will get a tasty performance boost. So roast some beets for dinner, and reserve one for smoothies. If you don't have time to roast beets, use canned beets instead.

- 1 small cooked beet (¼ c.), sliced
- ¾ cup frozen raspberries
- ½ cup orange juice
- 1 large pear, cored and sliced
- ½ serving vanilla whey protein powder

1 To cook beets: Preheat oven to 350 degrees F. Wash beets, cut off greens, and trim tips. Wrap in foil and place in a baking pan. Bake for about 1 hour or until you can easily pierce the cooked beets with a knife. Let cool until they can be handled, then peel away skin.

2 Combine all ingredients in blender and process until smooth.

Makes one 16-ounce smoothie.

Per serving: 286 calories, 3 g fat, 50 g total carbohydrate, 7 g dietary fiber, 12 g protein

DQS COUNT (per serving) FRUITS 1 VEGETABLES ½

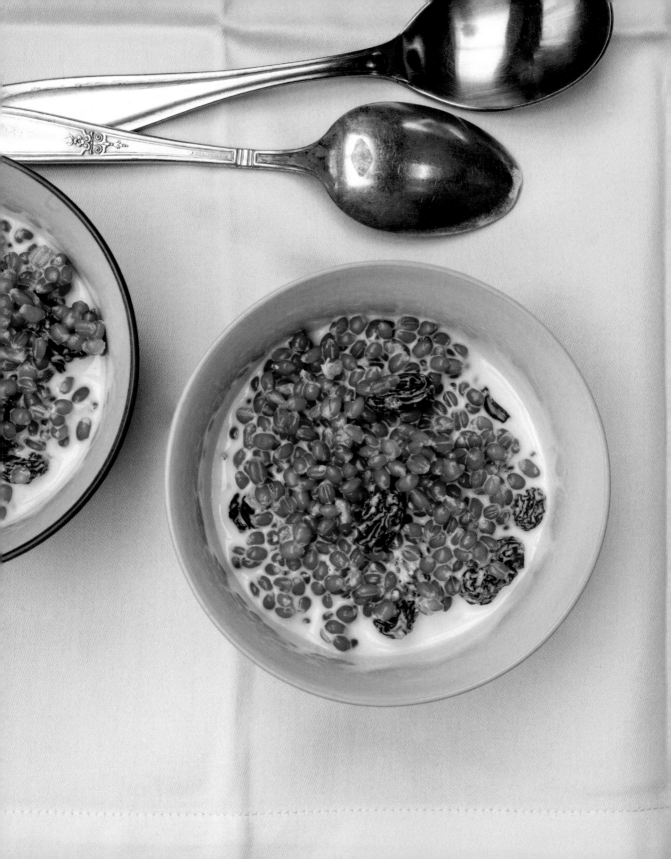

CINNAMON-RAISIN WHEAT BERRY BOWL

2 SERVINGS // 65 MINUTES

With steamed milk and the nutty aroma of toasted wheat berries, this breakfast cereal is worth the wait. If you have cooked wheat berries on hand, scoop 1½ cups into your pot, and wholesome goodness is just minutes away.

½ cup wheat berries, rinsed and drained

1½ cups water

1 cup 1% milk (or whole milk, soy, or almond milk)

¼ cup raisins

¼ teaspoon cinnamon

½ teaspoon vanilla extract (optional)

1 In a dry saucepan over medium heat, toast wheat berries for about 5 minutes, taking care to stir them with a wooden spoon so they brown and don't burn. Once you start to smell the aroma of the wheat berries, you will know that they are sufficiently toasted.

2 Add water to wheat berries and bring to a boil over medium-high heat. Cover and let simmer for 45 minutes, or until wheat berries reach the desired texture.

3 Drain any remaining liquid, then add milk, raisins, cinnamon, and vanilla, if desired. Stir frequently to keep milk from scalding. Continue cooking until milk begins to thicken and raisins become plump, about 5 minutes.

4 Divide between two bowls and top with an extra sprinkle of cinnamon.

Per serving: 300 calories, 3 g fat, 59 g total carbohydrate, 6 g dietary fiber, 12 g protein

DQS COUNT (per serving)   FRUITS ½   WHOLE GRAINS 1   DAIRY 1

PUMPKIN SPICE MUFFINS

12 SERVINGS // 40 MINUTES

Perfectly full of warm spices and pumpkin, these muffins are a real treat when paired with a steaming beverage on a crisp autumn day.

cooking spray

1½ cups whole-wheat flour

2 tablespoons ground flaxseed

1 teaspoon baking soda

½ teaspoon baking powder

1½ teaspoons cinnamon

1 teaspoon ground cloves

½ teaspoon each ground nutmeg, allspice, and ginger

½ teaspoon salt

¾ cup sugar

2 tablespoons canola oil

½ cup unsweetened applesauce

½ cup (4) egg whites or egg substitute

1 cup canned pumpkin puree

1 teaspoon vanilla extract

1 Preheat oven to 325 degrees F. Use cooking spray to lightly coat the 12 wells of a standard muffin tin. As an alternative, use silicone muffin molds, which do not need to be greased.

2 In a large bowl, combine flour, flaxseed, baking soda, baking powder, cinnamon, cloves, nutmeg, allspice, ginger, and salt.

3 In a second large bowl, blend together sugar, canola oil, applesauce, egg whites, pumpkin, and vanilla. Add to dry ingredients and stir just until uniformly moistened.

4 Divide batter between 12 muffin wells and bake for 25 minutes, or until tops spring back when lightly touched.

Wrap leftover muffins in plastic wrap. Refrigerate for up to one week, or freeze for up to six months.

Per serving: 145 calories, 3 g fat, 27 g total carbohydrate, 3 g dietary fiber, 4 g protein

DQS COUNT (per serving)   WHOLE GRAINS   1

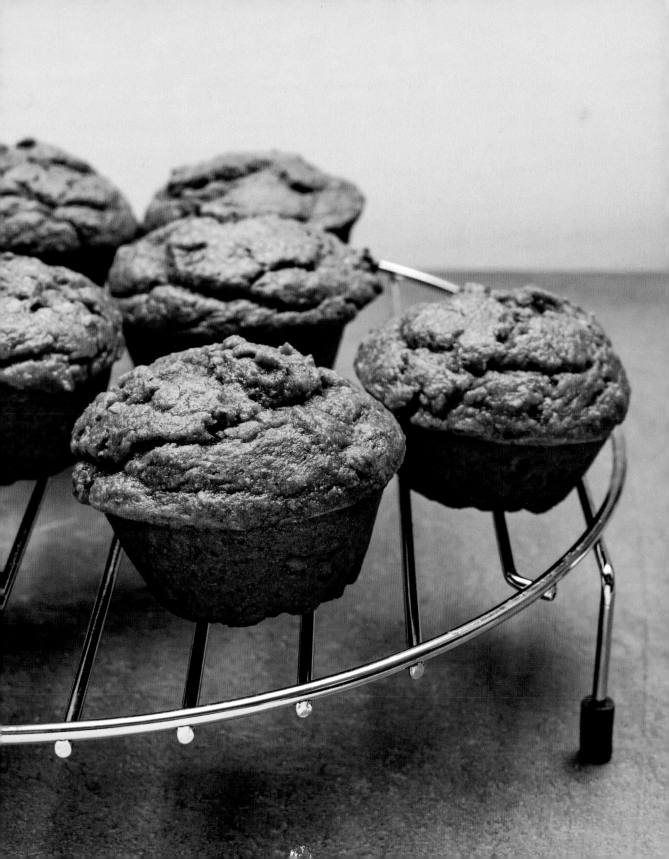

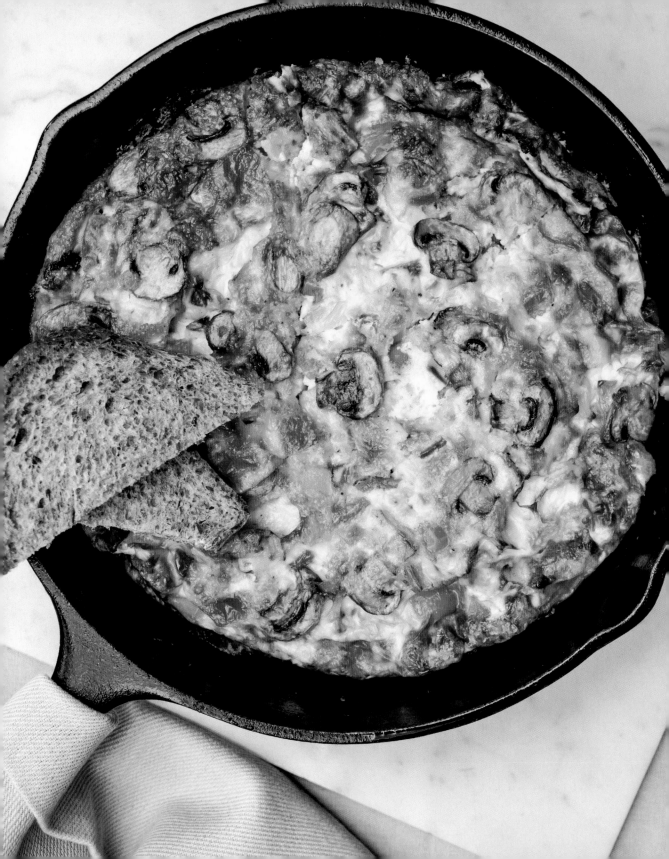

VEGETABLE FRITTATA

4 SERVINGS // 1 HOUR

1 teaspoon extra-virgin olive oil

1 cup mushrooms, sliced

1 cup green, red, and yellow peppers, chopped

1 cup onion, chopped

1 large tomato, chopped

4 eggs, beaten

2 cups egg substitute

1 cup (4 oz.) mozzarella cheese, cubed

¼ teaspoon salt

¼ teaspoon pepper

1 Preheat oven to 375 degrees F. Lightly coat a cast-iron or ovenproof skillet with olive oil.

2 Add mushrooms, peppers, and onion. Cook over medium-high heat until soft, then turn off heat.

3 In a large mixing bowl, combine tomato, eggs, egg substitute, cheese, and salt and pepper. Pour egg mixture into the skillet and stir a little to distribute vegetables and cheese evenly.

4 Bake for 45 minutes or until the center of the frittata is set and the color is golden brown.

Per serving: 227 calories, 11 g fat, 8 g total carbohydrate, 1 g dietary fiber, 25 g protein

SUNDAY CHOPFEST

With a busy weekday schedule, you might not want to bother chopping fresh vegetables for every meal. One option is to buy precut vegetables at the grocery store; but you'll spend a bit more for the convenience. To save money, you can set aside 20 to 30 minutes on Sunday and cut up vegetables to use all week. Make a big container of chopped mushrooms, peppers, and onions for easy omelets, or a bulk mix of peppers, onions, broccoli, and carrots for a quick stir-fry. Use containers with resealable lids or large plastic bags to keep odors from filling the whole fridge, and use your precut veggies within five days.

DQS COUNT (per serving)   VEGETABLES 1   LEAN MEATS & FISH 1   DAIRY 1

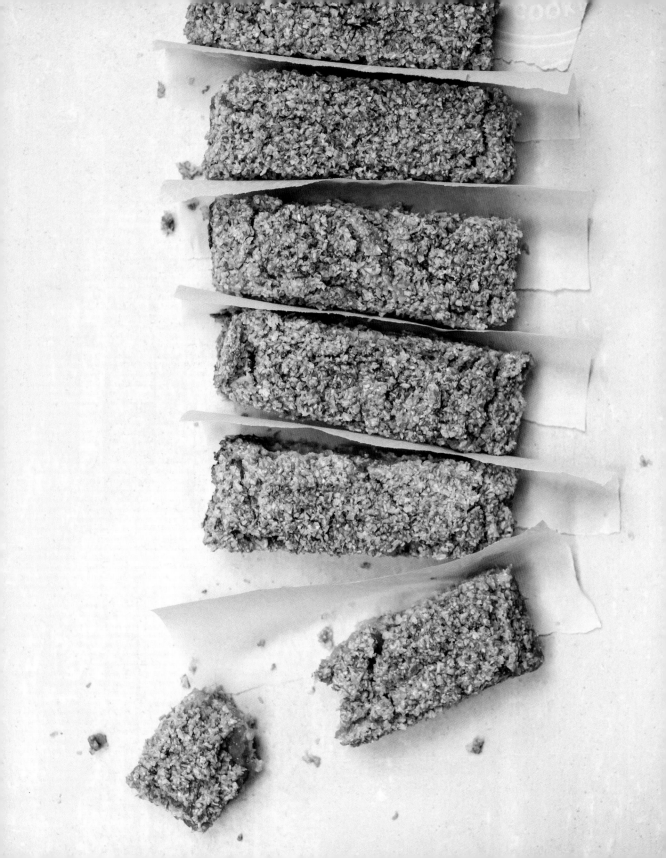

FIG & BRAN BARS

6 SERVINGS // 40 MINUTES

Perfect for stashing in lunch boxes and gym bags, these bars are made with wheat bran, oat bran, and 100% fig filling! The hearty texture and flavor make these bars a great high-carbohydrate snack after a workout. You can use either light- or dark-colored figs, or if you prefer, try unsulfured dried apricots for a different fruit flavor.

cooking spray

¾ cup (3 oz.) dried figs

1 cup water, divided

1 cup oat bran

½ cup wheat bran

2 tablespoons sugar

½ tablespoon baking powder

½ teaspoon salt

1½ tablespoons butter (room temperature)

1 egg

1 Preheat oven to 325 degees F. Line an 8 × 4-inch loaf pan with foil, letting some hang over the sides for easy removal after baking. Mist foil lining lightly with cooking spray.

2 Finely chop figs and place in a medium saucepan with ½ cup water. Bring to a simmer and cook for 5 minutes, stirring occasionally. Transfer mixture to blender and process until smooth.

3 In a large mixing bowl, combine oat bran, wheat bran, sugar, baking powder, and salt. Stir to blend. Add butter; work in with a rubber spatula until mixture is crumbly. Add egg and remaining ½ cup water, and stir just until dough comes together.

4 Spread half of dough evenly in the foil-lined pan. Top with fig mixture and smooth with rubber spatula. Top with remaining batter and smooth gently with rubber spatula.

5 Bake for 25 minutes. Cool completely before cutting into 6 bars.

Individually wrap leftover bars in plastic wrap. Store in refrigerator for up to one week or freeze.

Per serving: 164 calories, 5 g fat, 32 g total carbohydrate, 8 g dietary fiber, 5 g protein

DQS COUNT (per serving) FRUITS ½ WHOLE GRAINS 1

RASPBERRY SCONES

8 SERVINGS // 30 MINUTES

While the crumbly, slightly sweet taste of a good scone is not something I want to live without, typical coffee-shop scones are made with refined wheat flour and contain more sugar than you might think. These scones taste delicious and include higher-quality ingredients.

cooking spray

1¼ cup white whole-wheat flour

1 cup quick oats

¼ cup sugar

1½ teaspoons baking powder

¼ teaspoon baking soda

¼ teaspoon salt

¼ teaspoon cinnamon

¼ teaspoon ground ginger

5 tablespoons butter, melted

⅓ cup almond milk (or dairy)

1 teaspoon lemon juice

½ cup (4) egg whites

1 cup raspberries, fresh or frozen

1 Preheat oven to 400 degrees F. Use cooking spray to lightly coat a cast-iron scone pan. (You may also use a cookie sheet to make drop scones.)

2 In a large bowl, combine flour, oats, sugar, baking powder, baking soda, salt, cinnamon, and ginger and stir to mix well.

3 In a small bowl, mix melted butter, milk, lemon juice, and egg whites. Pour into bowl with dry ingredients and stir to mix. Gently fold in raspberries and spoon batter into scone pan or drop in 8 equal mounds on a cookie sheet.

4 Bake for 20 minutes or until tops and edges are golden brown. Allow scones to cool before removing from pan.

Per serving: 203 calories, 8 g fat, 26 g total carbohydrate, 4 g dietary fiber, 6 g protein

Try substituting blueberries or other types of fruit for raspberries.

DQS COUNT (per serving)   WHOLE GRAINS   1

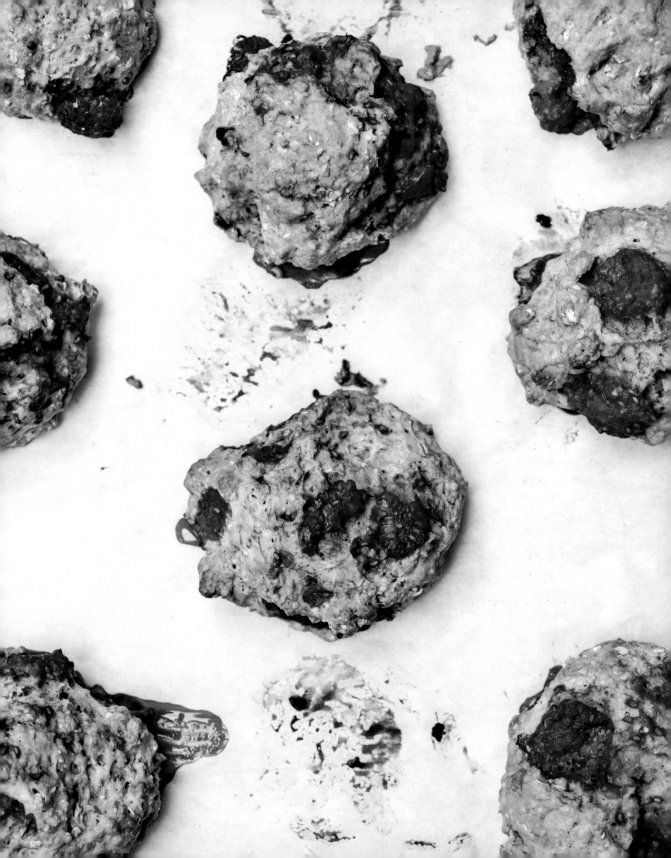

APPLE-RAISIN BARS

8 OR 12 SERVINGS // 35 MINUTES

Try these oat bars for a breakfast on the run or for postworkout refueling. Cut into 8 portions for meal-sized servings or 12 for snack-sized bars.

cooking spray

1½ cups quick oats

1 cup whole-wheat flour

3 servings (1 c.) vanilla whey protein powder

1 cup sugar

3 tablespoons ground flaxseed

1 tablespoon baking powder

1 teaspoon baking soda

1 teaspoon ground cinnamon

½ teaspoon salt

¾ cup nonfat plain Greek yogurt

½ cup (4) egg whites or egg substitute

¼ cup water

2 tablespoons canola or macadamia-nut oil

1 teaspoon vanilla extract

1 large apple, finely chopped

¼ cup raisins, not packed

1 Preheat oven to 350 degrees F. Spray a 9 × 13-inch baking dish with cooking spray.

2 In a large mixing bowl, combine oats, flour, whey protein, sugar, flaxseed, baking powder, baking soda, cinnamon, and salt. Stir to blend.

3 In a separate mixing bowl, combine yogurt, egg whites, water, oil, and vanilla. Stir in chopped apple and raisins. Add wet ingredients to bowl containing dry ingredients. Stir to blend just until uniformly moistened. Spread batter in pan.

4 Bake for 15–17 minutes until center is just solid; allow to cool completely before cutting into bars.

Wrap individually in plastic wrap and store in refrigerator or freezer.

Per serving (for 8 bars): 343 calories, 6 g fat, 57 g total carbohydrate, 5 g dietary fiber, 16 g protein

Per serving (for 12 bars): 275 calories, 5 g fat, 46 g total carbohydrate, 4 g dietary fiber, 13 g protein

DQS COUNT (per serving)   WHOLE GRAINS   1

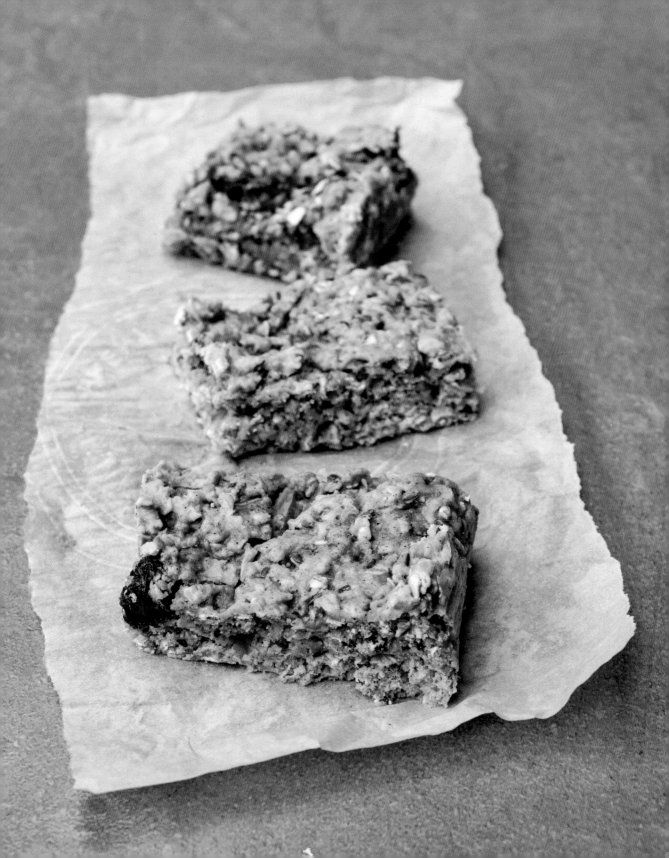

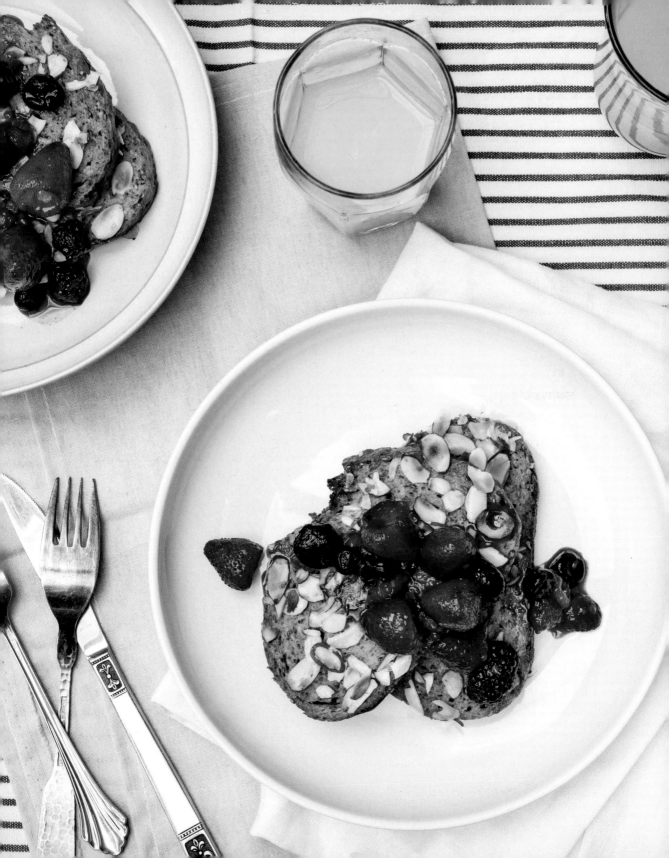

ALMOND-CRUSTED FRENCH TOAST WITH BERRIES

2 SERVINGS // 20 MINUTES

I like to use frozen berries in place of syrup for this French toast. As the berries defrost, they become more juicy. If you have fresh berries on hand, they will be just as nice.

2 eggs

¼ cup (2) egg whites

¼ cup milk or almond milk

1 teaspoon cinnamon

½ teaspoon vanilla extract

¼ cup sliced almonds

1 teaspoon butter

4 slices 100% whole-wheat bread

2 cups mixed berries (fresh or frozen)

1 In a wide, shallow bowl, combine egg, egg whites, milk, cinnamon, and vanilla and beat lightly with a fork to blend. Spread sliced almonds on a separate plate.

2 Heat a skillet over medium heat and melt butter. Place one piece of bread into egg mixture, and turn to coat both sides. Let excess egg drip away, then gently press each side into almonds. Place coated bread in the hot pan. Repeat process with remaining bread slices.

3 Cook for about 5 minutes on each side or until golden brown, then transfer to a plate to keep warm until serving.

4 If using frozen berries, microwave in a bowl for 2 minutes. Spoon berries over toast.

Per serving: 408 calories, 16 g fat, 44 g total carbohydrate, 11 g dietary fiber, 19 g protein

DQS COUNT (per serving)　FRUITS　1　WHOLE GRAINS　1　NUTS & SEEDS　½

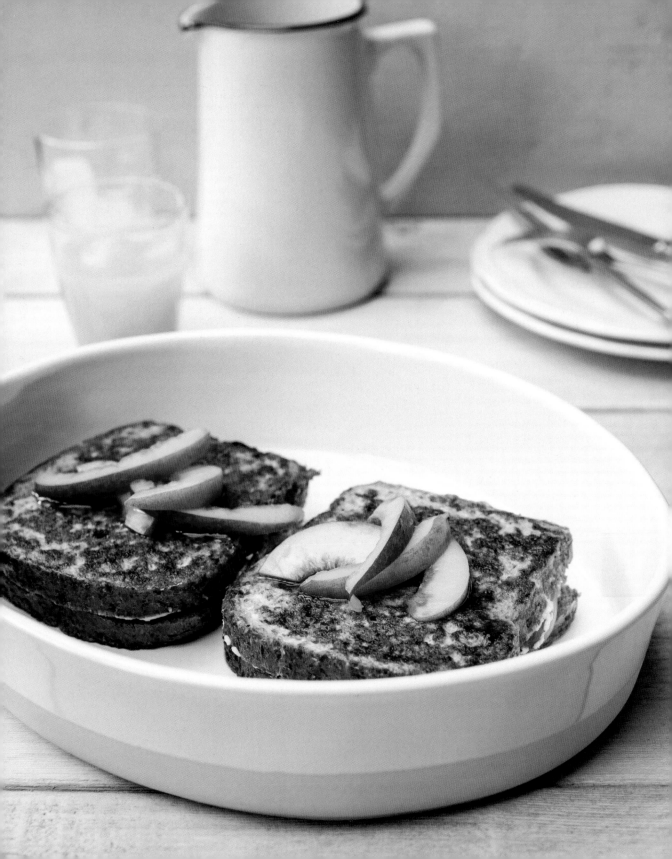

NECTARINE & SWEET CHEESE–STUFFED FRENCH TOAST

2 SERVINGS // 25 MINUTES

- 2 eggs, beaten
- 2 tablespoons milk (or almond milk)
- 1 teaspoon vanilla extract
- ½ cup ricotta cheese (regular or part skim)
- 3 teaspoons honey
- 4 slices whole-wheat or sprouted-grain bread
- 2 nectarines, thinly sliced
- 2 teaspoons butter, divided
- 1 tablespoon maple syrup (or additional honey)

1 In a shallow, wide bowl, stir together eggs, milk, and vanilla. In a second bowl, stir together ricotta and honey.

2 Spread two slices of bread with ¼ cup ricotta mixture, and top with nectarine slices. Make into a sandwich. Repeat with the two remaining slices of bread. Place the sandwiches in the egg batter, let sit for a minute, and flip to soak the other side. Allow to sit longer, and turn again to soak up the egg mixture.

3 Melt 1 teaspoon butter over medium-low heat in a hot skillet. Place sandwiches in the pan and cover. Cook for 5 minutes, then remove lid and flip sandwiches. Replace lid and cook for 5 minutes longer. Transfer sandwiches to plate and cut on the diagonal. Cover to keep warm.

4 Add remaining 1 teaspoon butter, remaining nectarine slices, and maple syrup to pan. Cook for 3 minutes, then pour over stuffed French toast and serve.

Per serving: 510 calories, 16 g fat, 66 g total carbohydrate, 12 g dietary fiber, 26 g protein

For a smoother cheese filling, substitute 3 tablespoons light cream cheese for the ricotta.

DQS COUNT (per serving)　FRUITS　1　WHOLE GRAINS　1　DAIRY　½

SCRAMBLED EGGS
WITH CHEDDAR & APPLE

1 SERVING // 20 MINUTES

½ teaspoon extra-virgin olive oil

2 eggs

½ apple, chopped

2 tablespoons (½ oz.) cheddar cheese, grated

4 cups fresh spinach, loosely packed

1 red bell pepper, chopped

¼ onion, chopped

3 white or brown mushrooms

hot sauce

salt and pepper (optional)

1 Place a frying pan over low heat and add olive oil. As the pan warms, lightly beat eggs in a small bowl, then pour into skillet. Add apple and cook, stirring occasionally, until soft-scrambled. Sprinkle with cheese and turn off heat, but leave the skillet on the stovetop to keep warm.

2 In a separate pan, combine spinach, red pepper, onion, and mushrooms. Cover and cook until soft, about 5 minutes. Season to taste with hot sauce and salt and pepper, if desired. Serve alongside scrambled eggs.

Per serving: 375 calories, 16 g fat, 29 g total carbohydrate, 7 g dietary fiber, 23 g protein

 TIP

You can also use 5 ounces of frozen spinach—just thaw first.

DQS COUNT (per serving)   VEGETABLES   1   LEAN MEATS & FISH   1   DAIRY   ½

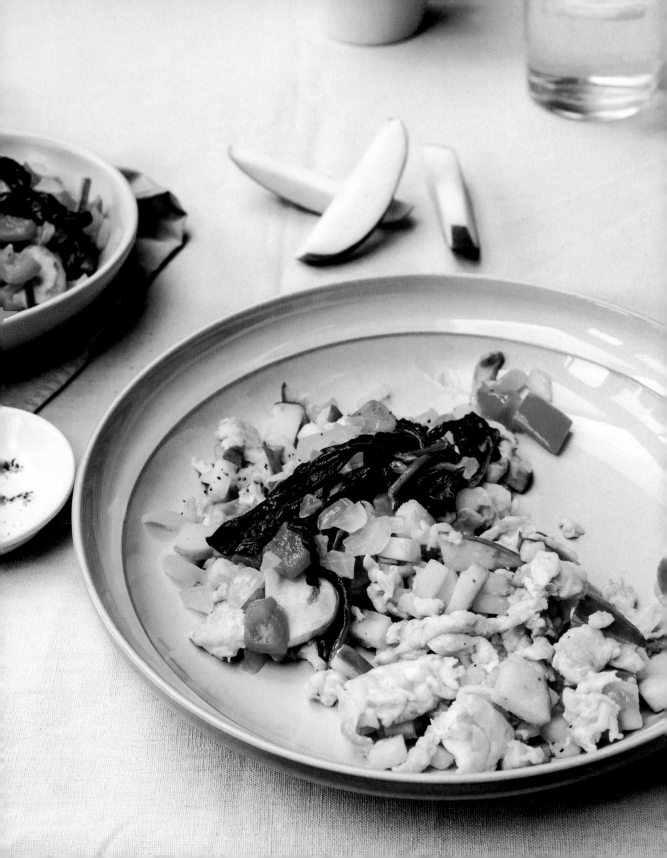

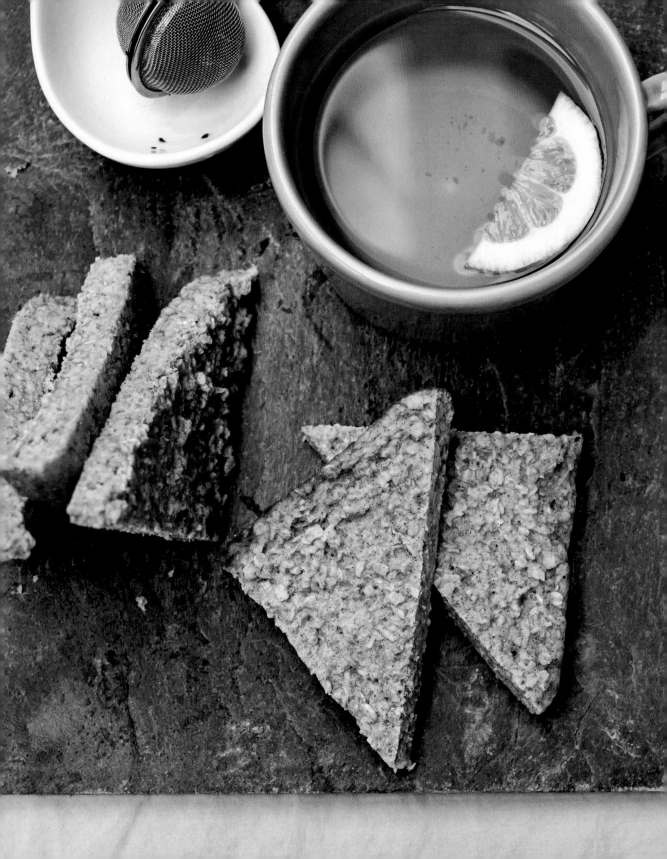

VANILLA-CHAI OATMEAL BARS

8 SERVINGS // 20 MINUTES

cooking spray

⅔ cup egg whites

½ cup plain nonfat yogurt

2 teaspoons vanilla extract

1 tablespoon canola oil

1½ cups quick oats

½ cup sugar

1½ teaspoons chai spice (see below)

½ teaspoon baking powder

¼ teaspoon salt

1 serving (⅓ c.) vanilla whey protein powder

CHAI SPICE

2 tablespoons ground cardamom

1 tablespoon ground cinnamon

1 teaspoon ground ginger

½ teaspoon ground cloves

½ teaspoon ground allspice

1 Preheat oven to 375 degrees F and lightly coat an 8-inch square pan with cooking spray.

2 In a small bowl, mix all chai ingredients together. Set aside.

3 In a large bowl, mix together egg whites, yogurt, vanilla, and oil. In a second bowl, combine remaining ingredients. Add wet ingredients to dry ingredients and stir until uniform.

4 Spread mixture evenly in prepared pan. Bake for 14 minutes. Cool and cut into 8 servings.

Store leftover chai spice in an airtight container or a plastic bag.

Per serving: 152 calories, 3 g fat, 24 g total carbohydrate, 2 g dietary fiber, 9 g protein

DQS COUNT (per serving)   WHOLE GRAINS   1

SPICED SWEET-POTATO & ALMOND SMOOTHIE

1 SERVING // 15 MINUTES PLUS 1 HOUR TO BAKE SWEET POTATO

1 medium sweet potato

1 cup unsweetened vanilla almond milk

1 tablespoon almond butter

1 serving vanilla protein powder

¼ teaspoon pumpkin-pie spice (plus extra for garnish)

1 Preheat oven to 400 degrees F. Wrap sweet potato in foil and bake for 60 minutes. Allow to cool before handling. May be prepared up to three days in advance.

2 Scoop ½ cup of flesh from sweet potato. (Refrigerate the remaining flesh for another smoothie, or freeze for longer-term storage.)

3 Place cooked sweet potato and all other ingredients in a blender. Process until smooth. Garnish with an extra sprinkle of pumpkin-pie spice.

Makes one 12-ounce smoothie.

Per serving: 320 calories, 11 g fat, 30 g total carbohydrate, 6 g dietary fiber, 25 g protein

+ CARBS Use 1 cup of sweet-potato flesh for a total of 51 g carbohydrate, and add 2 tablespoons of water if the smoothie is too thick. The color will be more orange.

DQS COUNT (per serving)   VEGETABLES 1   NUTS & SEEDS ½

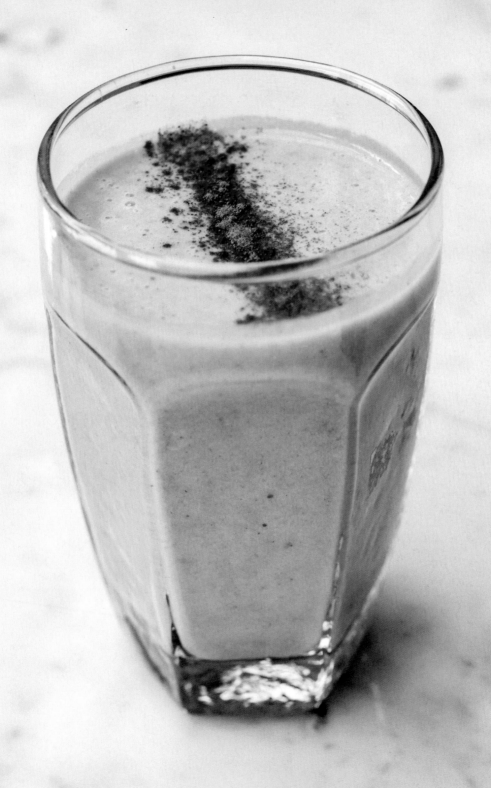

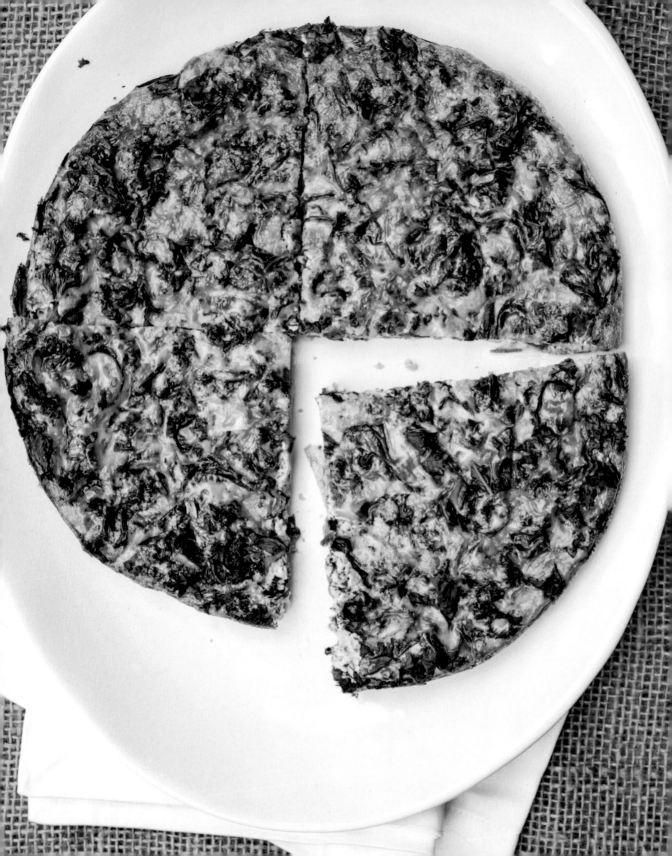

CRUSTLESS KALE QUICHE

4 SERVINGS // 1 HOUR (HP) (R) (V)

olive-oil cooking spray

1 bunch kale, stems removed, chopped

4 eggs

2 cups egg whites or egg substitute

1 cup (4 oz.) mozzarella cheese, shredded

½ teaspoon salt

¼ teaspoon black pepper

pinch of red pepper flakes (optional)

1 Preheat oven to 375 degrees F. Coat a cast-iron pan with cooking spray.

2 Place kale in pan and cook over medium heat, stirring occasionally, until tender, about 8 minutes. Turn off heat.

3 In a separate mixing bowl, combine eggs, egg substitute, cheese, salt, pepper, and red pepper flakes, if desired. Pour into skillet with kale and stir lightly to combine.

4 Bake for 45 minutes. Slice into 4 wedges.

Per serving: 246 calories, 11 g fat, 7 g total carbohydrate, 1 g dietary fiber, 25 g protein

DQS COUNT (per serving)   VEGETABLES ½   LEAN MEATS & FISH 1   DAIRY 1

BLUEBERRY SPELT QUICK BREAD

10 SERVINGS // 45 MINUTES

This lightly sweetened whole-grain loaf calls for spelt flour, which gives it a unique nutty flavor and lightness. You can also use whole-wheat flour, which works just the same in recipes. Grab a slice of this and add a smear of almond butter for a delicious speedy breakfast, or stash away a slice or two for a postworkout carb boost.

cooking spray

1¼ cups whole-grain spelt flour (or whole-wheat flour)

½ cup sugar

1½ teaspoons baking powder

½ teaspoon baking soda

½ teaspoon salt

1 tablespoon coconut oil or canola oil

½ cup unsweetened applesauce

2 eggs

1 cup fresh blueberries

1 Preheat oven to 325 degrees F. Lightly coat a loaf pan with cooking spray.

2 In a large bowl, combine flour, sugar, baking powder, baking soda, and salt and mix well.

3 In a second bowl, mix oil, applesauce, and eggs. Add the dry mix to the liquid ingredients, and stir just until everything is moistened. Fold in berries. Pour batter into prepared loaf pan.

4 Bake for 30–35 minutes, or until a knife inserted in the center comes out clean. Cool completely before slicing.

Store leftover slices in plastic bags in the refrigerator for up to one week, or stash them in the freezer for up to four months.

Per serving: 151 calories, 3 g fat, 29 g total carbohydrate, 3 g dietary fiber, 3 g protein

DQS COUNT (per serving)   WHOLE GRAINS   1

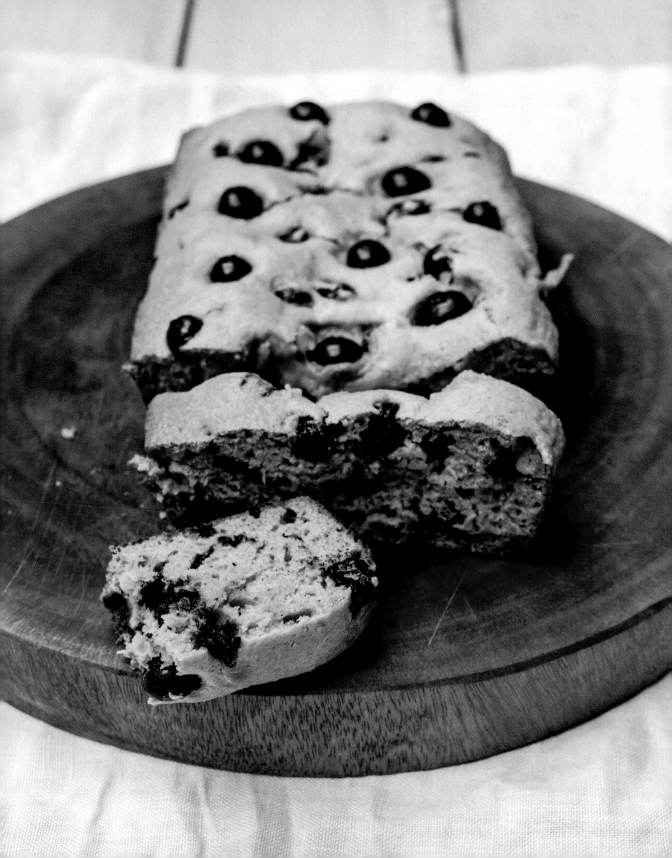

SAVORY ZUCCHINI PANCAKES

2 SERVINGS (2 PANCAKES) // 20 MINUTES

Pancakes don't have to be sweet. Top these savory pancakes with some crumbled cheese—feta, gorgonzola, or cotija will taste great. If you need more carbs, serve your pancakes with a generous helping of potatoes.

2 medium zucchinis

3 eggs

½ cup (4) egg whites or egg substitute

2 tablespoons coconut flour (or potato flour), rounded

½ teaspoon salt

black pepper

cooking spray

¼ cup cheese of your choice, shredded or crumbled

1 Use the fine side of a box grater to grate zucchini. Place grated zucchini in a large bowl and add remaining ingredients: eggs, flour, salt, and a generous grind of black pepper. Stir with a fork to break up any lumps.

2 Heat a 9-inch nonstick skillet over medium-low heat and coat lightly with cooking spray. When hot, add half of pancake mixture, making four small pancakes. Cover but leave lid ajar to vent steam. Cook until pancakes set, 5 minutes or a bit longer.

3 Flip pancakes and let them cook for a few minutes on the other side, then top with cheese. Cover for 1 minute if you want cheese to melt. Transfer to a plate, and repeat with the remaining batter. Stack pancakes onto two plates and dig in.

Makes 4 small pancakes.

Per serving: 286 calories, 15 g fat, 15 g total carbohydrate, 5 g dietary fiber, 26 g protein

(See **Homemade Turkey Sausage Patties** recipe on p. 202)

Take care not to overcook, as the eggs and zucchini will dry out. Your pancakes should still be soft to the touch.

DQS COUNT (per serving)   VEGETABLES 1   LEAN MEATS & FISH 1   DAIRY ½

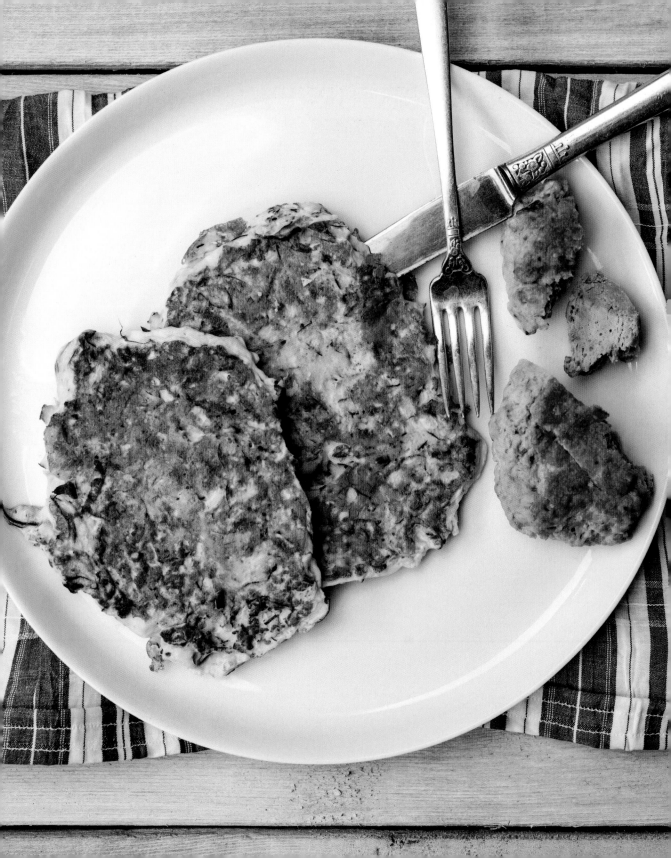

HOMEMADE TURKEY SAUSAGE PATTIES

12 SERVINGS (1 PATTY) // 30 MINUTES **HP** (See photo on p. 201)

Store these sausage patties in the freezer uncooked. I like to make them spicy. If you want the flavor to be more mild, decrease the cayenne and red pepper flakes.

1½ **pounds 93% lean ground turkey (or ground pork)**

½ **tablespoon dried rubbed sage**

1 **teaspoon dried thyme**

2 **teaspoons red pepper flakes**

½ **teaspoon cayenne pepper**

½ **teaspoon salt**

½ **teaspoon black pepper**

1 Place ground turkey in a large bowl. In a small bowl, mix together all the spices. Use your hands to blend the spices evenly into the meat.

2 Form 12 patties, placing them on layers of wax paper or parchment paper to keep them from sticking. I place two patties next to each other on each layer of parchment and stack them four or five high, then place the stack in an airtight plastic bag and freeze.

3 When breakfast time rolls around, take the desired number of sausage patties out of the bag and place in a pan. Cook over medium-high heat in a skillet for 4–5 minutes on each side or until cooked through.

Makes 12 2-ounce patties.

Per serving: 81 calories, 4 g fat, 0 g total carbohydrate, 0 g dietary fiber, 11 g protein

To test the seasoning, pinch off a small piece and cook in a pan to taste and see if it needs more salt, etc., or if you like it as is.

DQS COUNT (per serving) LEAN MEATS & FISH 1

A WELL-STOCKED FREEZER

At the end of a busy day or after a long workout, it's nice to have a healthy meal that you can simply heat and eat. The freezer is great for stashing away precooked meals and leftovers, but you can also save time and money by freezing some of the ingredients you use most often.

INGREDIENTS TO COOK & FREEZE	+ Breads + Cooked proteins (beef, chicken, or turkey) + Cooked whole grains (barley, quinoa, or wheat berries) + Vegetables to be cooked (either raw or blanched)
FOODS THAT FREEZE WELL	+ Baked goods (muffins & bars) + French toast + Pancakes + Pasta sauces + Soups
INGREDIENTS TO BUY FROZEN	+ Fruit (blueberries, cherries, mango chunks, or mixed berries) + Vegetables (bell-pepper strips, cauliflower, corn, pearl onions, or spinach) + Veggie burgers or vegetarian crumbles
FOODS THAT SHOULD NOT BE FROZEN	+ Cooked pasta + Roasted or well-cooked vegetables + Sauces with dairy or coconut milk + Vegetables you intend to eat raw

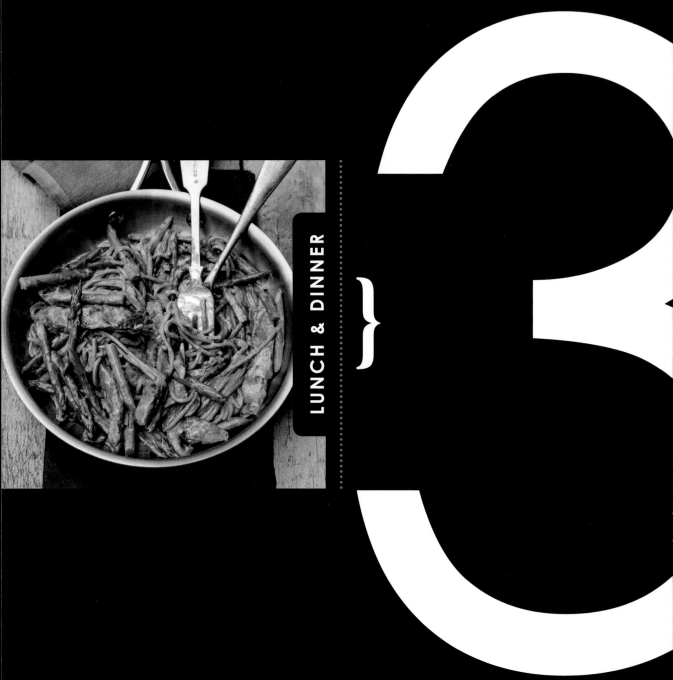

LUNCH & DINNER

3

THE ATHLETE WHO
LOVES TO COOK

CURRIED CHICKEN SALAD WITH PISTACHIOS

4 SERVINGS // 1 HOUR PLUS TIME TO CHILL

1 pound boneless, skinless chicken breasts	Bring a large pot of water to a boil over medium-high heat. Add chicken breast, cover, and simmer until cooked through, about 40 minutes. Drain and let meat cool.
⅓ cup 2% plain yogurt	
¼ teaspoon salt	As chicken cools, prepare dressing by stirring together yogurt, salt, curry powder, turmeric, and cinnamon in a large bowl. Add celery, carrot, red onion, and pistachios. Stir to blend.
¼ teaspoon curry powder	
⅛ teaspoon turmeric	
1 pinch of cinnamon	
1 cup celery, chopped	When chicken is cool, chop into cubes and fold into dressing and veggies until fully incorporated. Taste and add more salt if needed. Chill before serving.
⅓ cup carrot, chopped	
⅓ cup red onion, chopped	
¼ cup (1 oz.) shelled pistachios, chopped	Per serving: 189 calories, 4 g fat, 5 g total carbohydrate, 1 g dietary fiber, 28 g protein

DQS COUNT (per serving) VEGETABLES ½   LEAN MEATS & FISH 1   NUTS & SEEDS ½

CHICKPEA-FLOUR CRACKERS

2 SERVINGS // 25 MINUTES

cooking spray	Preheat oven to 325 degrees F. Line a small baking sheet with parchment paper and mist with cooking spray.
½ cup chickpea (garbanzo bean) flour	
½ teaspoon canola oil	Combine chickpea flour, canola oil, baking powder, and salt and stir to blend. Add water and mix to make a smooth batter.
¼ teaspoon baking powder	
⅛ teaspoon salt, plus additional	Scrape mixture onto parchment paper and spread thin. Try not to make the edges too thin, or they may burn. Sprinkle lightly with additional salt, dried onion, and poppy seeds. Bake for 7 minutes, then remove from oven and cut into squares with a sharp knife.
¼ cup water	
dried onion flakes	
poppy seeds	
	Bake for 5–6 minutes longer, or until edges begin to get golden brown. Remove from oven and allow to cool slightly. Test one to see if it's crispy; if not, return to oven for a few more minutes.
	Make a small batch—these are best fresh and crisp.
	Per serving: 104 calories, 2 g fat, 14 g total carbohydrate, 2 g dietary fiber, 6 g protein

DQS COUNT (per serving) VEGETABLES 1 (1 legume)

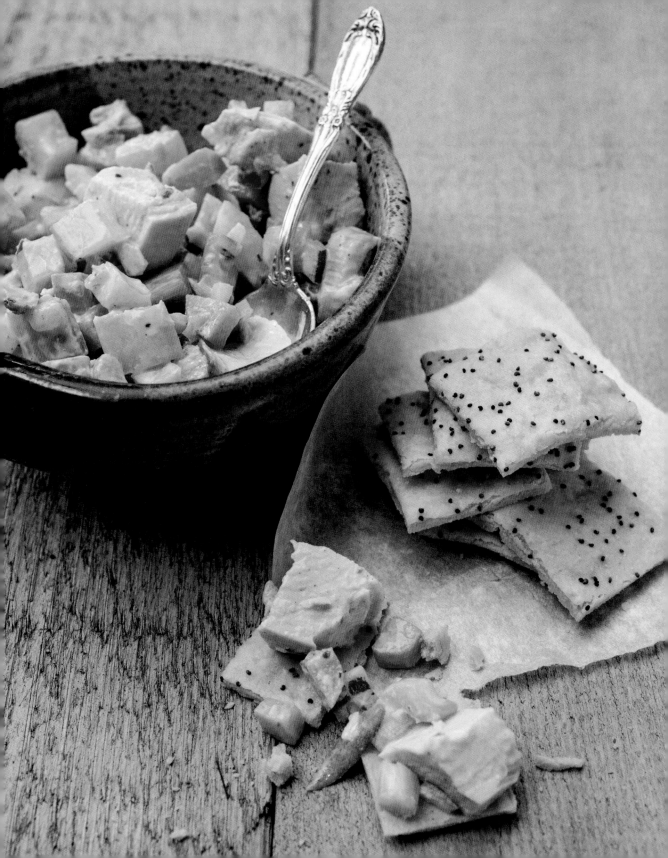

CARROT & CREMINI SOUP

2 SERVINGS // 40 MINUTES

This creamy soup gets its texture and sweetness from carrots and sour cream and is paired with the earthy flavor of sautéed mushrooms. If you can't get cremini (also known as baby bella) mushrooms, use another kind. Likewise, if you don't have a shallot on hand, use ⅛ of an onion.

4 cloves garlic

1 pound carrots, sliced

4½ cups vegetable broth

¼ cup sour cream

1 teaspoon extra-virgin olive oil

1 teaspoon butter

8 ounces cremini mushrooms, sliced

1 large shallot, halved lengthwise and sliced

salt and pepper

1 Combine garlic, carrots, and broth in a pot and bring to a boil. Reduce heat to medium and simmer for 30 minutes or until carrots are very tender.

2 Transfer mixture to blender and add sour cream. Cover and puree until completely smooth. Return to pot and keep warm over low heat.

3 In a medium pan, combine oil and butter over medium-high heat and then add mushrooms and shallot. Sprinkle lightly with salt and pepper to taste. Cook, stirring, over low heat for 10–15 minutes, until mushrooms are browned and soft.

4 Stir mushroom mixture into carrot soup and serve hot.

Per serving: 246 calories, 10 g fat, 32 g total carbohydrate, 8 g dietary fiber, 4 g protein

DQS COUNT (per serving)   VEGETABLES 2   DAIRY ½

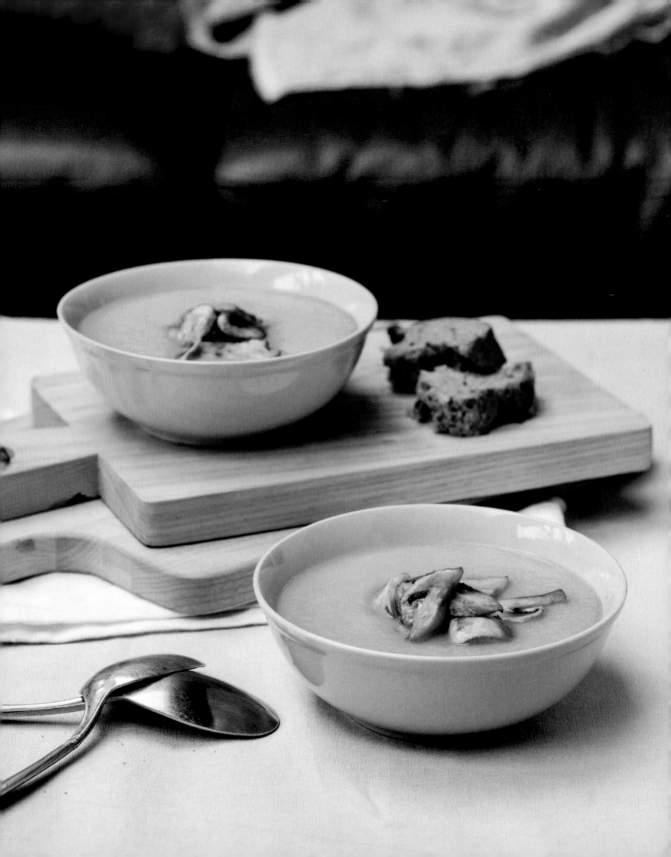

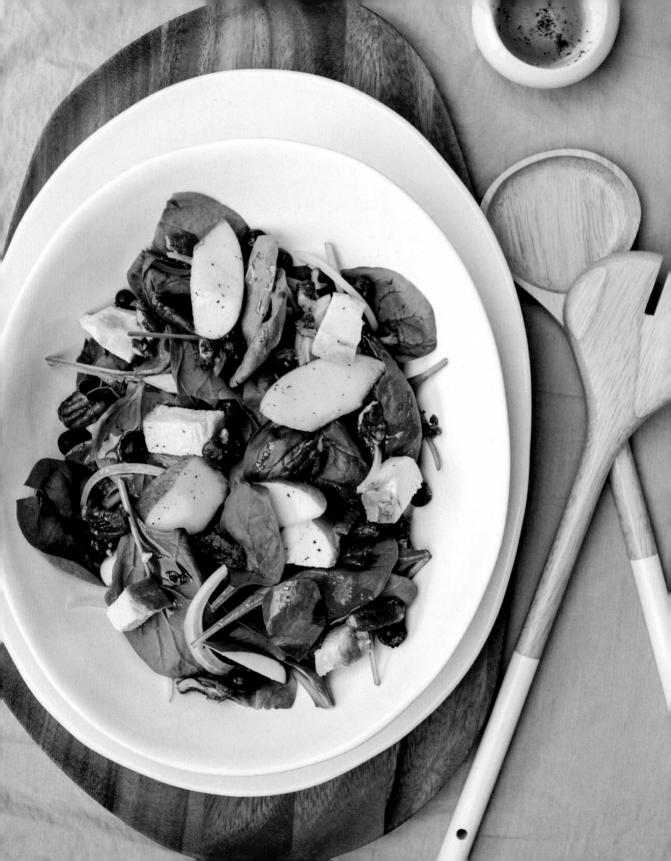

APPLE, BLUEBERRY & CHICKEN SALAD

2 SERVINGS // 10 MINUTES

6 cups (5 oz.) fresh baby spinach, loosely packed

¼ cup onion, sliced

2 teaspoons extra-virgin olive oil

1 tablespoon red wine vinegar

1½ cups *cooked* chicken breast, cubed

½ medium apple, diced

½ cup blueberries

In a large mixing bowl, combine spinach, onion, oil, and vinegar. Toss to mix.

Divide between two plates and top each salad with chicken, apple, and blueberries.

*Serve with ¼ cup **Fast & Easy Glazed Pecans** (recipe below).*

Per serving: 376 calories, 17 g fat, 18 g total carbohydrate, 6 g dietary fiber, 36 g protein

DQS COUNT (per serving) FRUITS 1   VEGETABLES 1   LEAN MEATS & FISH 1

FAST & EASY GLAZED PECANS

6 SERVINGS (2 TABLESPOONS) // 20 MINUTES

1 teaspoon butter

1 teaspoon honey

¾ cup (3 oz.) unsalted pecans (whole or pieces)

⅛ teaspoon cinnamon

⅛ teaspoon cayenne (optional)

pinch of salt

In a 10-inch skillet, combine butter and honey over medium heat. When mixture bubbles, turn heat down to low and cook for 1 minute. Add pecans and sprinkle with cinnamon and cayenne, if desired. Stir, and continue to cook on low for 5 minutes.

Turn off heat and sprinkle with salt. Allow pecans to cool and dry completely, about 10 minutes. Store leftovers in a plastic bag or jar.

Per serving: 109 calories, 11 g fat, 3 g total carbohydrate, 2 g dietary fiber, 1 g protein

Putting the pan into the freezer will dry the pecans quickly, but first allow the pan to cool for 5 minutes so that you won't melt the other items in your freezer.

DQS COUNT (per serving) NUTS & SEEDS ½

SEARED TUNA WITH MANGO-CUCUMBER SALSA

2 SERVINGS // 20 MINUTES

Searing the outside of the tuna showcases the natural beauty and tender texture of sushi-grade fish. The mango-cucumber salsa pairs well with any firm, flavorful fish.

8 ounces sushi-grade tuna

salt

freshly ground black pepper

1 teaspoon canola oil

MANGO-CUCUMBER SALSA

½ cup mango, finely chopped

½ cup cucumber, finely chopped

1 teaspoon lime juice

⅛ teaspoon salt

1 To make salsa, in a small bowl stir together mango, cucumber, lime juice, and salt. Set aside.

2 Season both sides of tuna with salt and pepper to taste. Place oil in medium nonstick skillet and heat over medium-high heat. When oil is very hot, add tuna and cook 1 minute on each side, or to desired level of doneness.

3 Remove from heat and cut into thin slices. Serve with mango-cucumber salsa.

Per serving: 183 calories, 4 g fat, 10 g total carbohydrate, 1 g dietary fiber, 27 g protein

+ CARBS Serve each portion with 1 cup cooked brown rice for 56 g total carbohydrate.

DQS COUNT (per serving)   FRUITS ½   LEAN MEATS & FISH   1

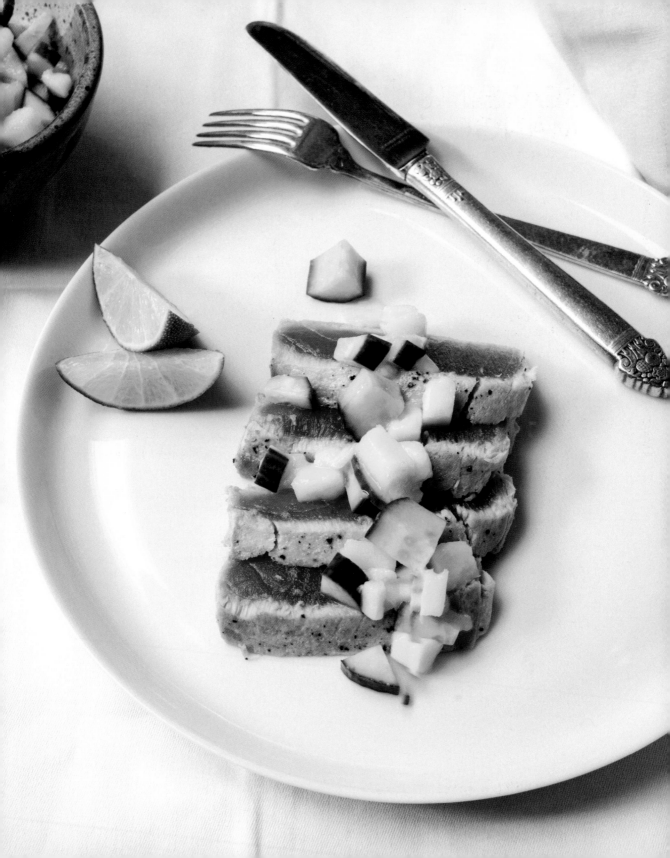

AUTUMN STUFFED ACORN SQUASH

4 SERVINGS // 45 MINUTES

Oven-roasted vegetables offer great flavor if you have the time to cook them. In a crunch, you can cook the squash in the microwave. Simply cover with damp paper towels to trap the steam and cook for 5 minutes or until tender.

2 acorn squash (about 1 lb. each)

2 teaspoons extra-virgin olive oil

¼ onion, chopped

1 pound boneless, skinless chicken breast, cubed

½ pear, chopped

6 white mushrooms, chopped

¼ cup (1 oz.) walnuts or pecans, chopped

¼ teaspoon each salt, cinnamon, allspice, and dried sage

⅛ teaspoon black pepper

1 Preheat oven to 375 degrees F. Cut the two squash into halves and scrape out the seeds. Place cut-side down in a glass dish with ½ inch water. Bake for 30 minutes, or until squash is tender.

2 Meanwhile, heat oil in a large nonstick skillet; add onion and chicken breast. Cook over medium heat, stirring every few minutes, for 8 minutes or until chicken is cooked through.

3 Add pear, mushrooms, walnuts, and seasonings. Cover the skillet with a lid and turn heat to low. Cook for 5 minutes, then turn off heat.

4 When the squash is finished baking, stuff each half with the chicken-and-pear filling.

Per serving: 284 calories, 8 g fat, 27 g total carbohydrate, 4 g dietary fiber, 26 g protein

DQS COUNT (per serving) | VEGETABLES 1 | LEAN MEATS & FISH 1 | NUTS & SEEDS ½

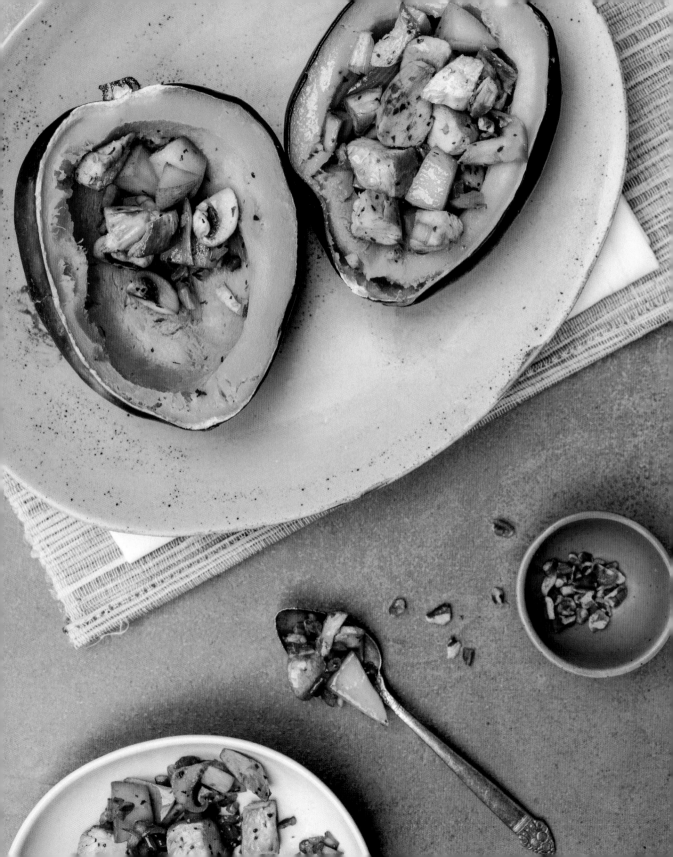

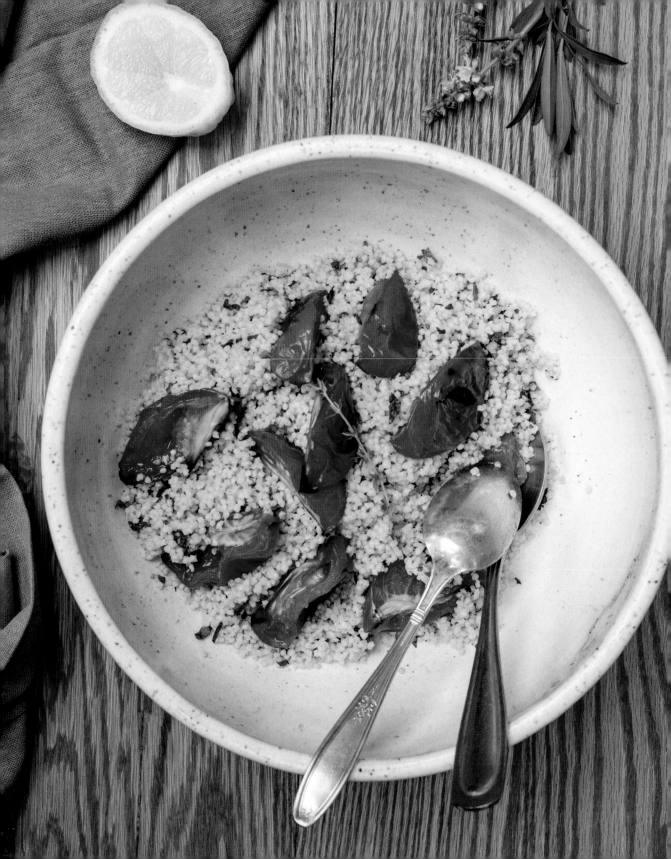

MILLET WITH HERBS & ROASTED TOMATOES

4 SERVINGS (1 CUP) // 40 MINUTES

Millet is a gluten-free whole grain that is a delicious alternative to nutty-flavored quinoa. Millet has a lighter, more delicate flavor, similar in taste to white rice but far more nutritious. It can be substituted for quinoa in recipes with no adjustments to cooking time or liquid.

6 Roma or plum tomatoes

2 cups water

1 cup millet, rinsed and drained

½ cup mixed fresh parsley, cilantro, and dill, loosely packed

1 tablespoon lemon juice

1 tablespoon extra-virgin olive oil

¼ teaspoon salt

⅛ teaspoon black pepper

1 Preheat oven to 500 degrees F. Line a baking sheet with foil. Quarter tomatoes and place skin-side up on baking sheet. Bake for 30 minutes.

2 Meanwhile, bring 2 cups water to a boil in a medium saucepan. Stir in millet. When water returns to a boil, reduce heat to low, cover, and simmer for 12 minutes. Turn off heat and steam with the cover on for 5 more minutes.

3 Finely chop parsley, cilantro, and dill. Stir chopped herbs, lemon juice, olive oil, and salt and pepper into millet.

4 When tomatoes have finished roasting, they should have some blackened spots. If not, broil them for an additional 5 minutes. Then gently fold them into millet.

Per serving: 282 calories, 7 g fat, 48 g total carbohydrate, 6 g dietary fiber, 7 g protein

DQS COUNT (per serving)   VEGETABLES 1   WHOLE GRAINS 1

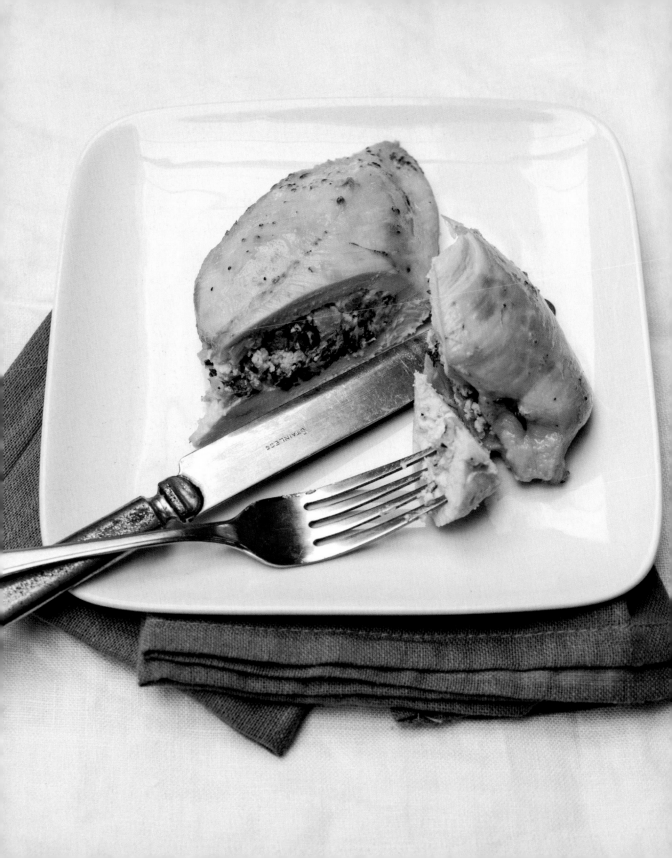

APRICOT, BASIL & GOAT CHEESE–STUFFED CHICKEN

4 SERVINGS // 45 MINUTES

olive-oil cooking spray

10 large fresh basil leaves, shredded

4 dried apricots, finely chopped

¼ cup (2 oz.) goat cheese, crumbled

⅛ teaspoon salt, plus additional

⅛ teaspoon black pepper, plus additional

1¼ pounds boneless, skinless chicken breasts

1 Preheat oven to 400 degrees F and line a baking sheet with parchment paper. Lightly coat with olive-oil cooking spray and set aside.

2 In a medium bowl, combine basil, apricots, goat cheese, salt, and pepper.

3 Place chicken on a cutting board and use a paring knife to slice the side of each chicken breast to create a pocket to hold the filling. Enlarge the pocket carefully without cutting all the way through. Divide filling between pieces of chicken.

4 Lightly season outside of stuffed chicken with additional salt and pepper. Place on prepared sheet and cover with foil. Bake for 30 minutes, then remove foil and broil for 3 minutes to brown surface.

Per serving: 195 calories, 5 g fat, 5 g total carbohydrate, 2 g dietary fiber, 34 g protein

+ CARBS Serve each portion with 1 cup **Millet with Herbs & Roasted Tomatoes** (p. 217) for 53 g total carbohydrate.

DQS COUNT (per serving) LEAN MEATS & FISH 1   DAIRY 1

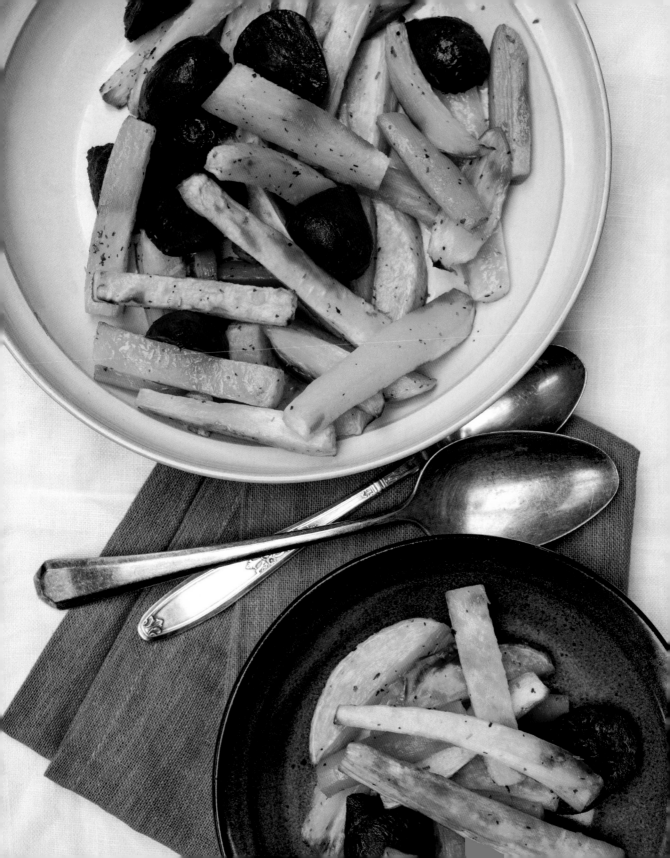

ROOT VEGETABLES
WITH ROSEMARY & OLIVE OIL

4 SERVINGS // 50 MINUTES

This rainbow dish is both stunning and delicious. I've listed the weights as purchased, which will be slightly less after trimming.

8 ounces beets (without tops)

8 ounces parsnips

8 ounces carrots

8 ounces rutabaga

1 yellow onion

1½ tablespoons extra-virgin olive oil

1 tablespoon fresh rosemary leaves

seasoned salt

black pepper

1 Preheat oven to 425 degrees F.

2 Cut beets in half. Place flat-side down, and cut into slices about ⅓ inch thick. Place in a big mixing bowl.

3 Cut ends off parsnips, carrots, rutabaga, and onion and cut into ½-inch-wide strips. Add to the mixing bowl.

4 Add oil to the vegetables, and toss to coat. Spread veggies out on a cookie sheet and sprinkle with rosemary. Season lightly with seasoned salt and pepper to taste.

5 Bake for 30 minutes, and then check for doneness. Vegetables may need an additional 10–15 minutes to become tender.

Per serving: 148 calories, 5 g fat, 25 g total carbohydrate, 7 g dietary fiber, 2 g protein

DQS COUNT (per serving)   VEGETABLES   1

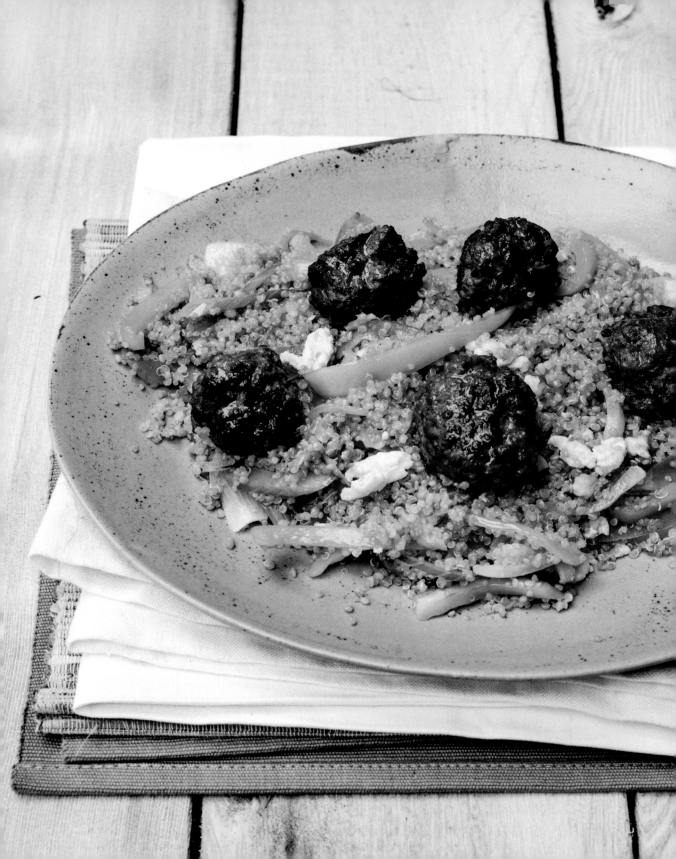

QUINOA "FRIED RICE"

4 SERVINGS (1¼ CUPS) // 30 MINUTES

- ¾ cup quinoa, rinsed and drained
- 1½ cups water
- 1 egg, beaten
- 1 teaspoon sesame oil
- ½ red pepper, chopped
- ½ yellow onion, chopped
- 2 celery ribs, chopped
- 1 clove garlic, crushed or minced
- 2 teaspoons soy sauce

Combine quinoa and water in a small saucepan and bring to a boil. Reduce heat to low and cover. Cook 20 minutes or until all water is absorbed, then turn off heat. Let quinoa cool, uncovered. (This lets extra moisture evaporate so the quinoa is dry.)

In a large nonstick skillet, scramble egg over medium heat, breaking into small pieces. Transfer cooked egg to a small plate or bowl and return skillet to stove.

Raise heat to medium-high and add sesame oil to skillet. Heat oil for 1 minute, then add red pepper, yellow onion, celery, and garlic. Stir-fry for 5 minutes, then add cooked quinoa, egg, and soy sauce. Cook, stirring for 2 minutes or until hot, and serve.

Per serving: 173 calories, 5 g fat, 27 g total carbohydrate, 4 g dietary fiber, 7 g protein

DQS COUNT (per serving)   VEGETABLES ½   WHOLE GRAINS 1

WASABI MEATBALLS

4 SERVINGS (8 MEATBALLS) // 30 MINUTES

- 1 pound 96% lean ground beef
- 3 cloves garlic, crushed or minced
- 1 tablespoon prepared wasabi paste
- 1 tablespoon soy sauce
- ½ teaspoon ground ginger
- ¼ teaspoon red pepper flakes

In a large mixing bowl, combine all ingredients and mix well. Form meat mixture into 32 1-inch meatballs, ½ ounce each.

Place meatballs in a single layer in a large nonstick skillet and cook over medium heat, turning occasionally, to brown outsides.

Cover skillet and reduce heat to low, cooking for an additional 10–15 minutes.

Per serving: 157 calories, 5 g fat, 3 g total carbohydrate, 1 g dietary fiber, 24 g protein

DQS COUNT (per serving)   LEAN MEATS & FISH 1

SPINACH & FETA PIE
WITH CHICKPEA-FLOUR CRUST

6 SERVINGS // 50 MINUTES

This pie makes a fabulous breakfast, lunch, or dinner, and it's just as good cold as it is hot—that is, really, really good!

cooking spray

1 pound *frozen* cut leaf spinach, thawed, moisture squeezed out

2 eggs

¾ cup (6 oz.) feta cheese, crumbled

½ cup 2% cottage cheese

¼ teaspoon salt

black pepper

CHICKPEA-FLOUR CRUST

1 cup chickpea flour (also called garbanzo-bean flour or besan)

1 tablespoon extra-virgin olive oil

¾ teaspoon salt

1 cup water

1 Preheat oven to 500 degrees F. Use cooking spray to lightly mist a cast-iron skillet; place skillet in oven and heat for at least 10 minutes.

2 In a large mixing bowl, whisk together crust ingredients, chickpea flour, olive oil, salt, and water, until there are no lumps.

3 Remove hot skillet from oven. Pour batter for crust into skillet. Return to oven for 10 minutes.

4 In a separate bowl, combine spinach with eggs, feta, cottage cheese, and salt. Blend well.

5 Remove skillet from oven, and reduce oven temperature to 400 degrees F. Spread spinach filling evenly over crust, sprinkle with black pepper, and bake for 20 minutes longer. Cool for 10 minutes before slicing into 6 pieces.

Per serving: 187 calories, 9 g fat, 13 g total carbohydrate, 5 g dietary fiber, 15 g protein

DQS COUNT (per serving)   VEGETABLES 1   DAIRY 1

SALMON CAKES

2 SERVINGS (3 CAKES) // 25 MINUTES

These flavorful patties may be served over steamed or sautéed cabbage or bok choy or with rice.

- 2 5-ounce cans boneless, skinless pink salmon
- 3 green onions, thinly sliced
- 1 tablespoon ginger, minced
- 2 teaspoons garlic, minced
- ¼ teaspoon salt
- ¼ cup whole-wheat panko crumbs (or breadcrumbs)
- 1 egg
- ½ teaspoon sesame oil

Combine salmon, green onions, ginger, garlic, and salt in a large bowl and mix well. Add panko crumbs and egg and mix gently to combine. Form into 6 cakes.

Heat sesame oil in a large skillet over medium heat. When hot, add salmon patties. Cook without disturbing for 4–5 minutes or until bottom is golden and crisp, then gently flip with a spatula and cook for an additional 4–5 minutes on other side.

Per serving: 248 calories, 9 g fat, 12 g total carbohydrate, 2 g dietary fiber, 30 g protein

+ CARBS Serve each portion over 1 cup **Wild Rice with Onion & Thyme** for 47 g total carbohydrate.

DQS COUNT (per serving)   LEAN MEATS & FISH   1

WILD RICE WITH ONION & THYME

4 SERVINGS (1 CUP) // 1 HOUR, 10 MINUTES

Wild rice has a rich, nutty flavor that's anything but boring.

- 4 cups water
- 1 cup wild rice, rinsed and drained
- 2 teaspoons extra-virgin olive oil
- 1 yellow onion, chopped
- 2 teaspoons dried thyme leaves
- ¼ teaspoon salt
- ⅛ teaspoon black pepper

Boil water in a saucepan and add rice. When mixture returns to a boil, reduce heat to low and cook for 45–60 minutes, depending on desired firmness (longer cooking results in softer grains, whereas shorter cooking time leaves them chewy). Drain excess water.

Heat oil in a large nonstick skillet and add onion and thyme. Cook over medium-low heat for 5–6 minutes or until onions are translucent. Stir cooked rice into onion-thyme mixture and add salt and pepper. Stir to blend.

Makes 3–4 cups.

Per serving: 174 calories, 3 g fat, 33 g carbohydrate, 3 g fiber, 6 g protein

DQS COUNT (per serving)   WHOLE GRAINS   1

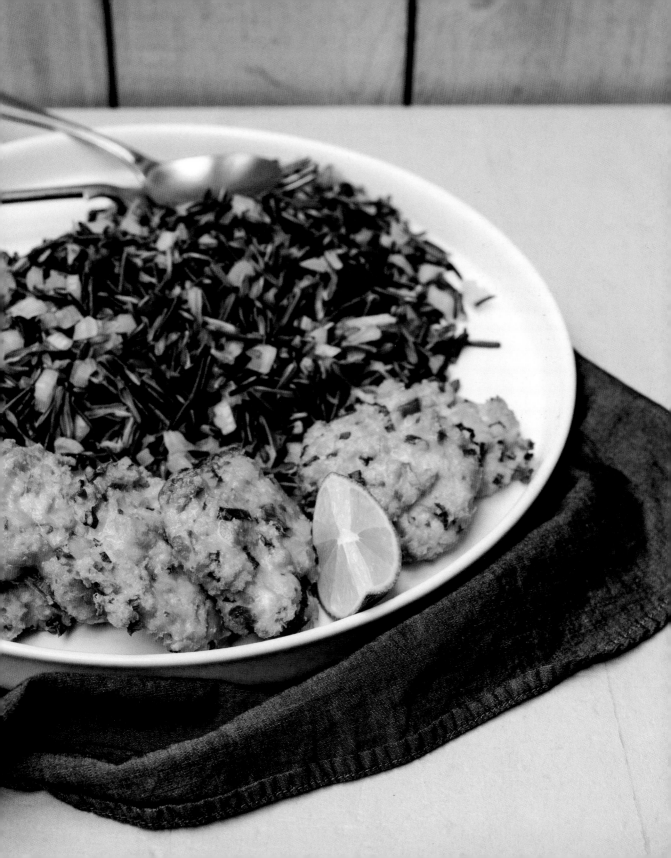

SOBA NOODLES WITH BEEF, ASPARAGUS & MUSHROOMS

2 SERVINGS // 25 MINUTES

4 ounces buckwheat soba noodles

cooking spray

4 cloves garlic, crushed

6 ounces lean beef, cut into strips

1 pound (1 bunch) asparagus, ends trimmed, cut into 3-inch pieces

2 cups mushrooms, sliced

2 tablespoons Thai red curry paste

4 teaspoons soy sauce or fish sauce

⅔ cup coconut milk

sriracha sauce

1 Bring a large pot of water to a boil and add soba noodles. Cook for 6 minutes, then drain in a colander and rinse with cold water.

2 Lightly coat a large skillet with cooking spray. Add garlic and beef and cook over medium heat for 2 minutes.

3 Add asparagus and mushrooms, stir, and cover. Cook for 4 minutes to steam vegetables lightly, then add curry paste, soy sauce, and coconut milk and stir to blend.

4 Add soba noodles and stir until noodles are evenly coated. Cook until sauce is reduced, about 5 minutes. Add sriracha sauce to taste to reach desired level of heat.

Per serving: 539 calories, 17 g fat, 58 g total carbohydrate, 5 g dietary fiber, 40 g protein

DQS COUNT (per serving) VEGETABLES 1 WHOLE GRAINS 1 LEAN MEATS & FISH 1

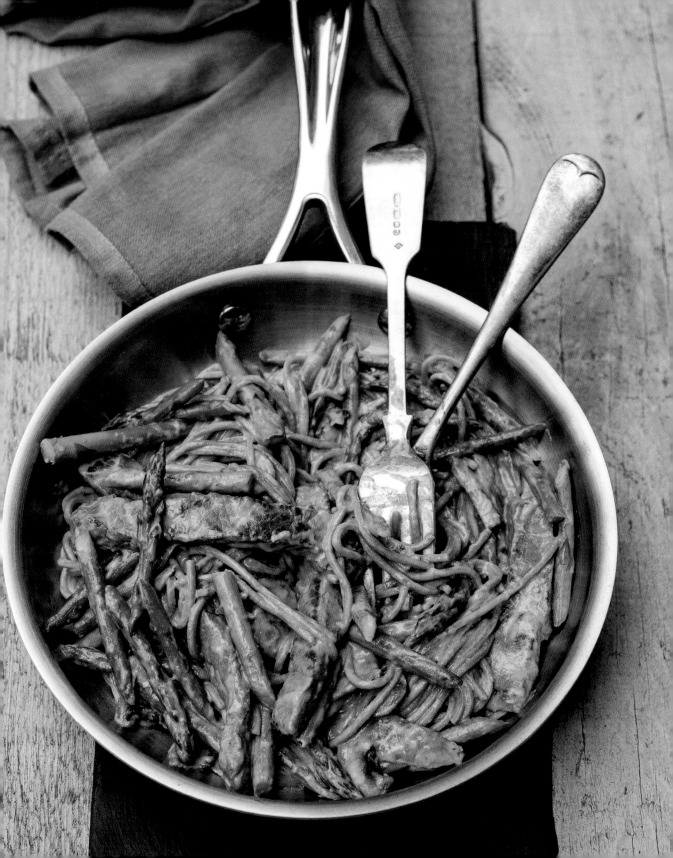

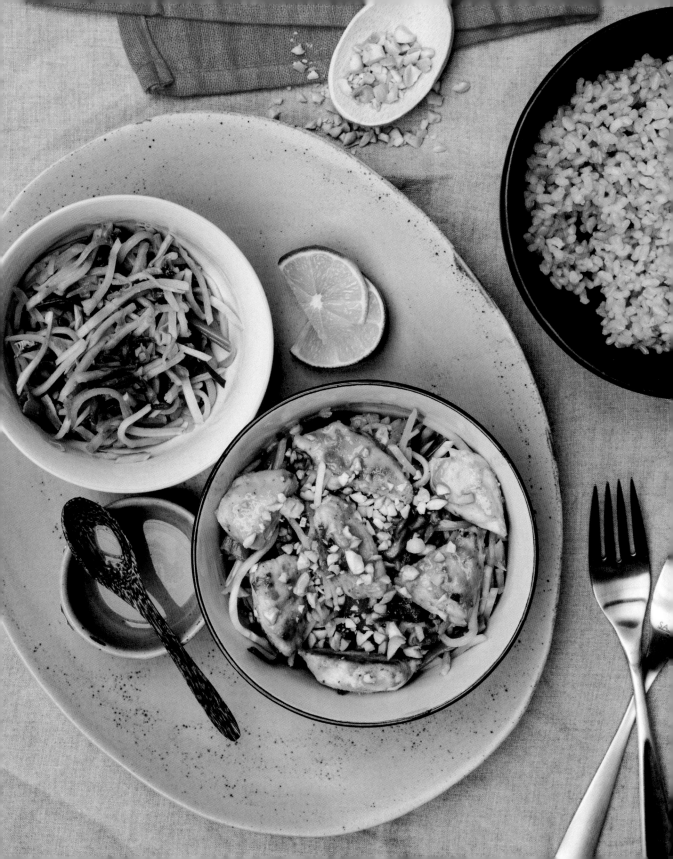

ASIAN CHICKEN WITH PEANUT SAUCE

3 SERVINGS // 20 MINUTES

This peanut sauce gets a low-fat makeover thanks to peanut flour, but you can use peanut butter if you don't have peanut flour on hand.

- 2 green onions, cut into 2-inch pieces
- 5 cups vegetables of your choice, julienned
- 1 pound boneless, skinless chicken breasts, cut into 2-inch pieces
- 3 cloves garlic, minced
- 2 tablespoons peanuts, chopped

PEANUT SAUCE

- 1 cup chicken broth
- ¼ cup peanut flour (or 2 tbsp. natural peanut butter)
- 1 tablespoon sriracha sauce
- 1 tablespoon honey
- 2 teaspoons soy sauce

1 In a small saucepan over low heat, combine all sauce ingredients. Stir and bring to a simmer. Keep simmering over low heat while preparing rest of meal, at least 2 minutes.

2 In a large nonstick skillet, combine onions, julienned vegetables, and ½ cup peanut sauce. Cook over medium-high heat until vegetables are tender and sauce is absorbed, 5–8 minutes. Transfer to serving dish and cover to keep warm.

3 Return pan to stove, and add chicken, garlic, and 2 tablespoons peanut sauce. Cook over medium-high heat until chicken is cooked through.

4 Serve chicken over vegetables, and spoon remaining peanut sauce over all. Garnish with chopped peanuts.

Per serving (with peanut flour): 312 calories, 4 g fat, 20 g total carbohydrate, 7 g dietary fiber, 45 g protein

Per serving (with peanut butter): 342 calories, 9 g fat, 20 g total carbohydrate, 6 g dietary fiber, 44 g protein

+ CARBS Serve over 1 cup cooked brown rice for 52 g total carbohydrate.

 TIP

Save time by using broccoli slaw (preshredded broccoli, cabbage, and carrots) in place of julienned vegetables. You can find it near bagged greens in most grocery stores.

DQS COUNT (per serving)   VEGETABLES 1   LEAN MEATS & FISH 1   NUTS & SEEDS ½

THAI GREEN CURRY WITH SHRIMP & SCALLOPS

4 SERVINGS // 25 MINUTES

1 teaspoon extra-virgin olive oil

2 tablespoons curry paste

2 tablespoons fish sauce

1 tablespoon brown sugar

1 red bell pepper, cut into strips

1 yellow bell pepper, cut into strips

½ red onion, sliced

3 white mushrooms, sliced

½ pound shrimp, peeled and deveined

½ pound bay scallops

2 plum tomatoes, chopped

1 cup coconut milk

1 Place oil and curry paste in a large nonstick skillet and heat on low for 5 minutes, stirring often. Add fish sauce and sugar; stir to dissolve sugar.

2 Add red pepper, yellow pepper, red onion, and mushrooms. Raise heat to medium and cook, stirring frequently, for 5 minutes.

3 Add shrimp, scallops, and tomatoes to skillet; reduce heat to low and add coconut milk. Stir continuously for 10 minutes, or until shrimp are opaque and scallops are firm. Mixture should steam but not come to a boil.

4 Remove from heat and divide among four bowls.

Per serving: 301 calories, 12 g fat, 26 g total carbohydrate, 4 g dietary fiber, 21 g protein

+ CARBS Serve with 1 cup brown rice for 58 g total carbohydrate.

DQS COUNT (per serving) VEGETABLES 1 LEAN MEATS & FISH 1

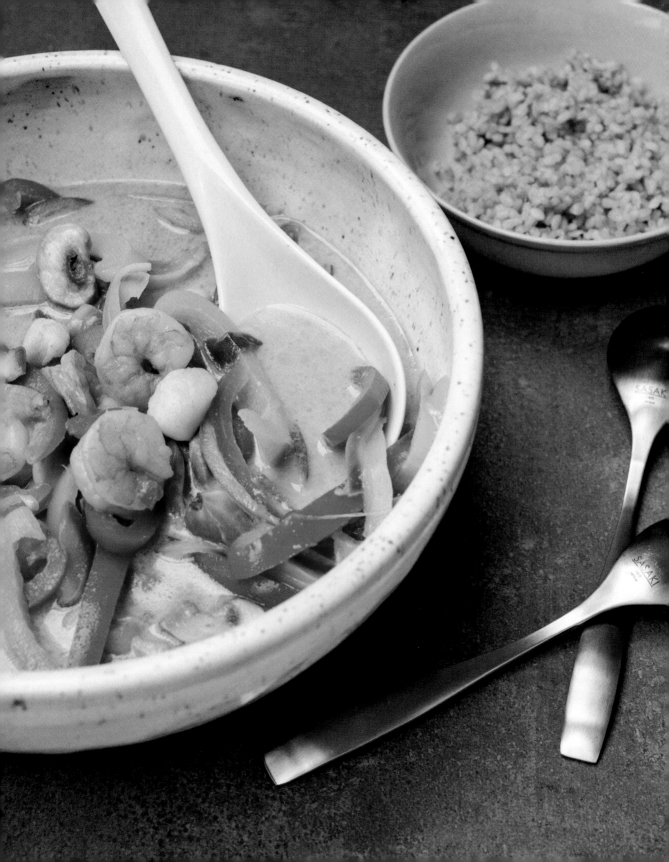

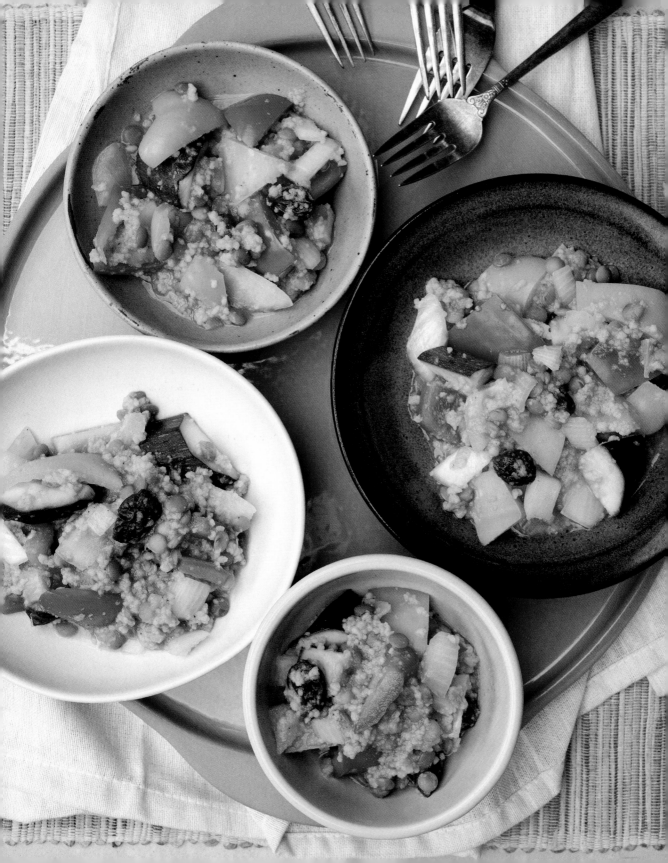

CURRIED LENTILS & COUSCOUS

4 SERVINGS // 30 MINUTES

This combination of lentils, couscous, vegetables, and seasonings provides slow-digesting carbohydrates and fiber, protein, and a slew of antioxidants from turmeric and bell peppers. A few plump raisins provide a pleasant hint of sweetness.

⅔ cup brown
   or green lentils

⅔ cup whole-wheat
   couscous

4 cups water

2 red bell peppers,
   seeded and chopped

2 yellow bell peppers,
   seeded and chopped

½ sweet onion, chopped

2 zucchinis, chopped

2 tablespoons (½ oz.)
   dark or golden raisins

2 teaspoons madras
   curry powder

1 teaspoon salt

½ teaspoon turmeric

1 Combine lentils, couscous, and water in a medium pot and bring to a boil. Reduce heat to low (do not cover), and set a timer for 20 minutes.

2 When 3 minutes remain on the timer, add peppers, onion, and zucchinis to the pot with raisins, curry powder, salt, and turmeric. Stir to blend.

3 Stir gently for the last 3 minutes, or until all liquid is absorbed.

Per serving: 262 calories, 1 g fat, 52 g total carbohydrate, 13 g dietary fiber, 14 g protein

DQS COUNT (per serving) VEGETABLES 1½ (½ legumes) WHOLE GRAINS 1

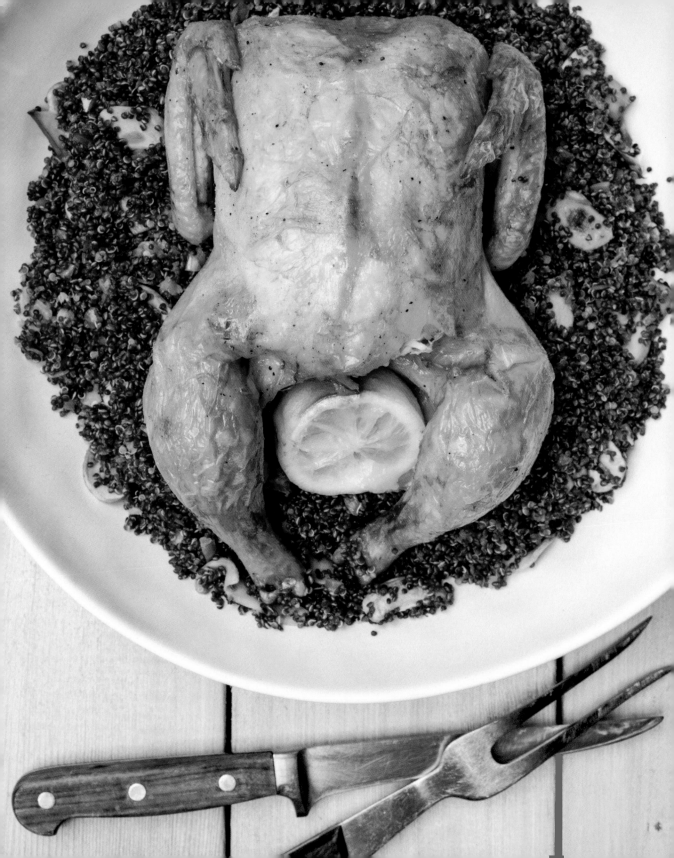

ROASTED CHICKEN

6 SERVINGS // 1 HOUR, 10 MINUTES

Roasting a whole chicken allows something for everyone: dark meat, white meat, and plenty of delicious leftovers! A meat thermometer is the safest way to tell when it's done before it dries out.

1 whole chicken
  (about 4 lbs.)

½ lemon

  salt, pepper,
  garlic powder

1 Preheat oven to 450 degrees F. Rinse chicken and pat dry with a paper towel. Place in roasting pan breast-side up, and squeeze juice from lemon over chicken, then place lemon inside cavity. Sprinkle chicken with salt, pepper, and garlic powder to taste.

2 Roast for 50–65 minutes or until thermometer inserted in thickest part of meat registers 165 degrees F. When chicken is done, remove from oven and let sit for 5 minutes before carving.

Per serving (without skin): 185 calories, 7 g fat, 0 g total carbohydrate, 0 g dietary fiber, 28 g protein

(See **Mushroom Quinoa** recipe on p. 238)

DQS COUNT (per serving)   LEAN MEATS & FISH   1

MUSHROOM QUINOA

6 SERVINGS // 35 MINUTES (See photo on p. 236)

- 1 tablespoon extra-virgin olive oil or butter
- 2 large shallots, sliced
- 3 cups mushrooms, sliced
- ¾ teaspoon salt
- 1½ cups quinoa
- ¼ teaspoon dried thyme
- 3 cups water

1 Place olive oil or butter in a saucepan over low heat. When melted, add shallots and cook until transparent. Add mushrooms and cook until soft and brown. Add salt, quinoa, and thyme, and stir to mix. Raise heat to medium and cook dry for 3–4 minutes to toast and heighten flavors.

2 Add water, stir, and bring to a boil, then reduce heat to low and simmer, covered, for 15 minutes. Turn off the heat, fluff quinoa with a fork, and allow it to sit, covered, for an additional 10 minutes to steam.

Per serving: 207 calories, 4 g fat, 34 g total carbohydrate, 4 g dietary fiber, 7 g protein

DQS COUNT (per serving) WHOLE GRAINS 1

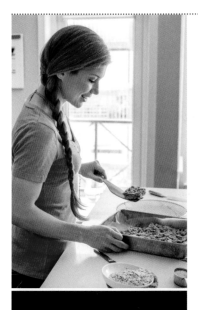

SMART TIPS FOR FOOD STORAGE

With some modest changes to how and where you store groceries, you can improve your diet quality and reduce food waste. When you open your refrigerator or pantry, you are more likely to eat the food that is most prominently placed. Reorganize your refrigerator to make the healthy foods more visible and accessible:

+ Keep fresh produce at eye level. Placing fruit and vegetables in the bins or drawers moves the healthiest choices out of sight and increases the odds that they'll spoil before you get around to using them. Prepare fresh-cut fruit and vegetables and store in clear plastic wrap or bags, ready for snacking.

+ Use the crisper drawers for things with a longer shelf life, such as cheese and yogurt.

+ Store raw meat and eggs on the bottom shelf, where they'll stay colder and be less likely to contaminate other foods.

+ Use aluminum foil or opaque containers for high-calorie items such as leftover pizza or restaurant foods.

If you do have processed or sweet foods on hand, tuck them away on the top shelf of the pantry. As an alternative, place a well-stocked fruit bowl on the kitchen counter or table.

ACKNOWLEDGMENTS

More than any other, this book is one that I could not have created alone. I am extremely grateful to Georgie Fear for the knowledge, experience, creativity, and energy she brought to this project. We are very fortunate to share the same first-class literary agent, Linda Konner. The dedicated staff at VeloPress did a remarkable job of transforming the raw materials we provided into an inviting and supremely useful final package. Peter Bagi's photography is so good you can almost taste it.

My most personal thanks go to my wife, Nataki, for helping me test the wonderful recipes in this book and to my mother, Laurie Fitzgerald, for those early cooking lessons that seemed so futile at the time.

Matt Fitzgerald

This cookbook would never have been born without Matt Fitzgerald's work to bring its predecessor, *Racing Weight*, to the bookshelf, and I'll always be grateful for the proposal to do this project together. It was fun from start to finish! I am grateful not only for Matt's ultrapractical style and clear prose but also for how he communicates in all his writing what the nutrition industry needs more of: evidence-based advice.

Thank you to my fine agent, Linda Konner; to Connie Oehring and Renee Jardine at Velo-Press for their tireless work to bring together a beautiful, organized book; and to Peter Bagi for his amazing food styling and photography.

To my incredible husband, Roland Fisher: Thanks for your constant support and understanding and for sharing life, love, and lots of meals with me.

Georgie Fear

CREDITS

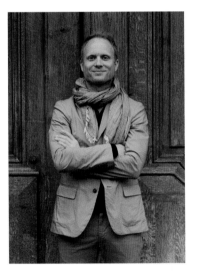

The world presents itself to me in the small details, and it's those details that I love to capture. I thrive in the simplicity that my best work comes from. Food is a natural choice for me to photograph, as I love to eat, cook, and share fantastic food experiences.

—Peter Bagi, photographer

Front cover, food, and Georgie Fear photographs; food prep & styling;
    prop styling: **Peter Bagi, www.peterbagi.com**
Assistant stylist: **Talia Harmuth**
Location 1: **home of Donna Seedorf-Harmuth and Phil Harmuth**
Location 2: **home of Veronique DaSilva**
Make-up stylist for Georgie Fear: **Erin Bradley**

Back cover photograph: **Matthias Robl**
Runner: **Jonathan Wyatt**

Matt Fitzgerald photographs: **Tom Hood**
Make-up stylist for Matt Fitzgerald: **Paula Serrano**

Cover design: **Samantha Jordan**
Art direction and interior design: **Vicki Hopewell**

Text set in Warnock and Haptic

DIET QUALITY SCORE TABLES

HOW TO SCORE YOUR DIET QUALITY

	FOOD TYPE	SERVING NUMBER					
		1st	2nd	3rd	4th	5th	6th
HIGH QUALITY	Fruits	2	2	2	1	0	0
	Vegetables	2	2	2	1	0	0
	Whole Grains	2	2	1	0	0	−1
	Lean Meats & Fish*	2	2	1	0	0	−1
	Nuts & Seeds	2	2	1	0	0	−1
	Dairy	1	1	1	0	−1	−2
LOW QUALITY	Refined Grains	−1	−1	−2	−2	−2	−2
	Fatty Proteins	−1	−1	−2	−2	−2	−2
	Sweets	−2	−2	−2	−2	−2	−2
	Fried Foods	−2	−2	−2	−2	−2	−2

* Plant proteins should be scored as vegetables if you are not a vegetarian.

HOW TO SCORE VEGETARIAN OR VEGAN DIETS

	FOOD TYPE	SERVING NUMBER					
		1st	2nd	3rd	4th	5th	6th
HIGH QUALITY	Fruits	2	2	2	1	0	0
	Vegetables	2	2	2	1	0	0
	Whole Grains	2	2	1	0	0	−1
	Legumes & Plant Proteins	2	2	1	0	0	−1
	Nuts & Seeds	2	2	1	0	0	−1
	Dairy	1	1	1	0	−1	−2
LOW QUALITY	Refined Grains	−1	−1	−2	−2	−2	−2
	Fatty Proteins	−1	−1	−2	−2	−2	−2
	Sweets	−2	−2	−2	−2	−2	−2
	Fried Foods	−2	−2	−2	−2	−2	−2

CONVERSIONS & EQUIVALENTS

EGGS

We use a mix of whole eggs and egg whites or egg substitute to keep recipes light. Equivalents are based on U.S. large eggs.

1 egg white = 2 tbsp.
4 egg whites = ½ c.
8 egg whites = 1 c.
1 egg = ¼ c. egg white or egg substitute

PROTEIN POWDER

If you don't have protein powder on hand, use flour as a substitute in baked goods.

1 serving = ⅓ c.

AMERICAN STANDARD VOLUME EQUIVALENTS

3 tsp. = 1 tbsp.
5 tbsp. + 1 tsp. = ⅓ c.
4 tbsp. = ¼ c.
8 tbsp. = ½ c.
16 tbsp. = 1 c.

IMPERIAL VOLUME EQUIVALENTS

1 tbsp. = ½ fl. oz.
2 tbsp. = 1 fl. oz.
1 c. = 8 fl. oz. (½ pint)
2 c. = 1 pint

METRIC VOLUME EQUIVALENTS

1 tsp. = 5 ml
1 tbsp. = 15 ml
¼ c. = 60 ml
½ c. = 125 ml
¾ c. = 175 ml
1 c. = 250 ml

METRIC WEIGHT EQUIVALENTS

1 oz. = 30 g
2 oz. = 60 g
4 oz. = 115 g
8 oz. = 225 g
1 lb. = 450 g
2 lb. = 900 g

NUTRIENT CONTENT GUIDE TO RECIPES

HC HIGH-CARBOHYDRATE RECIPES
(over 50 g carbohydrates)

BREAKFAST

Oat Bran with Cherries & Almonds, 41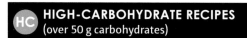

Tropical Mango Electrolyte Booster, 44 Ⓥ

Nut Butter & Banana Toast, 48 Ⓥ

Pumpkin & Maple-Nut Oatmeal, 102 Ⓥ

Coconut-Banana Protein Bars, 104 Ⓥ

Greena Colada Smoothie, 109 Ⓥ

Raspberry-Pear Smoothie, 173 Ⓥ

Cinnamon-Raisin Wheat Berry Bowl, 175 Ⓥ

Nectarine & Sweet Cheese–Stuffed French Toast, 189 Ⓥ

LUNCH & DINNER

Bean, Corn & Cheese Quesadilla, 59 Ⓥ

Tomato & Beef Florentine Soup, 63

Easy Eggplant Marinara, 67 Ⓥ

Garden Minestrone with Kale, 75 Ⓥ

Pork & Pepper Sauce over Rotini, 78

Brown Rice with Toasted Pine Nuts & Parmesan, 121 Ⓥ

Arugula, Barley & Blackberry Salad, 122 Ⓥ

Quinoa & Chickpea Salad, 130 Ⓥ

Turkey Meatballs & Fettuccine, 154

Greek Potatoes, 160 Ⓥ

Red Lentils with Kale & Tomatoes, 164 Ⓥ

Soba Noodles with Beef, Asparagus & Mushrooms, 228

Curried Lentils & Couscous, 235 Ⓥ

HIGH-CARBOHYDRATE STAPLES

Coupled with a main dish, these basic recipes have plenty of carbohydrates to fuel your training:

Basic Brown Rice, 120 Ⓥ

Garlic & Butter Brown Rice, 120 Ⓥ

Cilantro-Lime Brown Rice, 121 Ⓥ

Brown Rice with Toasted Pine Nuts & Parmesan, 121 Ⓥ

Millet with Herbs & Roasted Tomatoes, 217 Ⓥ

Wild Rice with Onion & Thyme, 226 Ⓥ

HP HIGH-PROTEIN RECIPES
(over 30% protein)

BREAKFAST

Toast with Cottage Cheese & Raspberry Preserves, 37 Ⓥ

Chocolate Chia Power Pudding, 43 Ⓥ

Hard-Boiled Eggs, 47 Ⓥ

Mushroom & Pepper-Jack Egg Muffins, 97 Ⓥ

Broccoli-Cheese Omelet, 107 Ⓥ

Greens, Eggs & Yam, 114 Ⓥ

Vegetable Frittata, 179 Ⓥ

Spiced Sweet-Potato & Almond Smoothie, 194 Ⓥ

Crustless Kale Quiche, 197 Ⓥ

Savory Zucchini Pancakes, 200 Ⓥ

Homemade Turkey Sausage Patties, 202

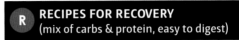

RECIPES FOR RECOVERY
(mix of carbs & protein, easy to digest)

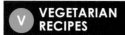

VEGETARIAN RECIPES

INDEX

Note: *Italic page numbers indicate photographs; t. indicates table. The numbers (1), (2), (3) following recipe titles indicate Levels 1, 2, or 3: (1) athlete who doesn't cook; (2) athlete with some cooking experience; (3) athlete who loves to cook.*

ABOUT THE AUTHORS

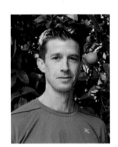

Matt Fitzgerald is an acclaimed endurance sports writer and authority. His many previous books for athletes include *Racing Weight* and *The New Rules of Marathon and Half Marathon Nutrition*. His writing has also appeared in magazines such as *Men's Journal*, *Outside*, and *Women's Running* and on competitor.com, active.com, and other websites.

A certified sports nutritionist, Matt has consulted for a number of sports nutrition companies and conducted peer reviews for scientific journals in the field. He currently serves as a training intelligence specialist for PEAR Sports. Matt has coached runners and triathletes since 2001 and continues to compete in running and multisport events, having started running at the age of 11. He lives in northern California with his wife, Nataki.

Georgie Fear is a professional nutrition coach whose advice is sought by athletes ranging from NCAA standouts to Olympic gold medalists. Her writing and recipes appear at askgeorgie.com and onebyonenutrition.com, and her recipe book, *Fuel Up* (2011), is available through Amazon.com.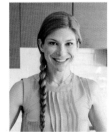

A registered dietitian and former rower, marathoner, and ultrarunner, Georgie has been helping clients get leaner, healthier, and faster since 2005. She previously worked as sports nutritionist for Rutgers University Athletics and presented her research and expertise at numerous nutrition and fitness conferences. She and her husband, Roland Fisher, currently own an Internet-based nutrition coaching company serving customers around the world. They live in Vancouver, British Columbia.

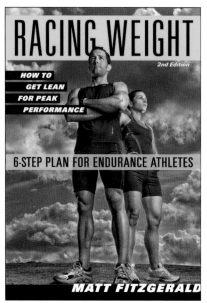
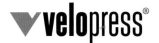